Playing in Traffic

AARON LIKENS

COASTAL181

CREDITS

Editing	*Bones Bourcier*
	Cary Stratton
Front Cover Photograph	*Walter Kuhn, IMS*
Back Cover Photograph	*Tony Leone*

Most of the photos in this book are from the Likens Family Collection. Every reasonable effort was made to locate and credit the original copyright holders and photographers of the other photos included on these pages. If your photo appears and you are not properly credited, please contact the publisher.

ISBN 13: 978-1-7362561-7-6

To request a speaking engagement, visit www.aaronlikens.com.

First printing April 2024

Published by:
Coastal 181
29 Water Street
Newburyport, MA, USA
877-907-8181
www.coastal181.com

Printed in the United States of America

PLAYING IN TRAFFIC
Table of Contents

─── **Dedication** ───

vii

For my dad, we did it!

To Duane, your flag set destiny in motion.

Foreword

I CAN'T REMEMBER IF I KNEW OF AARON LIKENS BEFORE I met him or, if after I met him, I told his story to so many people that it feels as if I have known him longer than I have. What I do remember, is seeing him flag the United States Auto Club Battle at the Brickyard event in the infield of IMS and learning that his desire was to one day stand in the flagstand overlooking the 2.5-mile historic oval and flagging the Indianapolis 500.

It was a lofty desire, wanting to flag the Indianapolis 500. Few have ever done it in the nearly 110 runnings of this historic race. And those that have, were icons of the sport. But something in the way Aaron talked to me about it, the way he understood what it meant, and how flagman Duane Sweeney had been his idol for so long, made me believe something from that moment … that one day, Aaron Likens would be the starter for the Indianapolis 500.

What I didn't know in the first meeting and what I learned over time was just how special a human Aaron Likens was, and is. He was passionate. He was professional. He was good under pressure. And managing a field of 33 race cars and drivers flashing beneath the flagstand at 240-plus miles per hour, in the largest sports stadium in the world, on the largest sports stage in the world, comes with pressure.

From his first introduction to the Indianapolis 500 as a young boy in 1989 and a souvenir checkered flag that went home with him that day, the path to the flagstand high above the finish line at Indianapolis was not easy. But the seeds that were sown that day would bear amazing fruit.

Challenges he faced discovering who he was, his "I wish …" papers, and his diagnosis of Asperger syndrome have all helped define and refine him along the way. One of Aaron's gifts has been that he has not let each challenge, each pain point, each struggle, slow him or defeat him. He has used those moments to spur him on, encourage him, and give him the personal green flag to go farther and reach higher.

Today, when you see Aaron in the flagstand, it is clear he belongs. His control of the situation and his use of his flags is a piece of art—created from years of building, learning, searching, and overcoming. There aren't many better stories and certainly not any better examples of inspiration than that of Aaron Likens.

So, in the words of my father, Jeff Boles—a long time racing official—who was in the flagstand the first time Aaron officially waived a flag over Indy Cars at IMS, welcome to *Playing in Traffic* authored by "Aaron Likens from St. Louis, Missouri. A tremendous starter in his own right." And, in my words, an even better person.

Green, green, green!

J. Douglas Boles
President
Indianapolis Motor Speedway

Playing in Traffic

IT'S SILENT. THERE ARE 135,000 PEOPLE AT THE Indianapolis Motor Speedway, but at this moment on the morning of May 30, 2021, there's no sound. I glance to my left and there's actor Milo Ventimiglia, here to throw the green flag as honorary race starter for the 105th running of the Indianapolis 500. To my right, there's a sea of people all the way to where the track curves out of sight. A bugle player from the 38th Infantry Division of the Indiana Army National Guard begins to play "Taps" in the official race flagstand directly above me, and I look up. The sun makes it hard to see, but I've had my eyes set on that stand for as long as I can remember.

And today is the day. I nearly say it out loud—"Today is the day!"—but I dare not speak during one of the most somber and eerily powerful moments in sports. However, realizing for the thousandth time what this day will bring has sent my pulse into a frenzy. I have never been more nervous. I feel truly alone in the middle of the largest public gathering since COVID-19 entered everyone's vocabulary.

The minutes are passing, and now Jim Cornelison is singing "Back Home Again in Indiana," a tradition on race day. I'm barely aware of it. I'm now within myself, trying to rationalize the moment. Achieving a life's goal is a rare achievement, and I'm about to become just the 11th person to hold the title of chief starter of the Indianapolis 500, the biggest automobile race in the world. That flagstand will be my post for the day.

~

When "Back Home" ended, a military flyover, the second of the day, roared overhead. I looked up, but my eyes were drawn across the track to the Tower Terrace grandstand and the section where I knew my dad was seated. I thought for a moment that I could almost make him out, or at least the hat he was wearing. This day, this phenomenal, improbable day for me, would not have been possible without my dad and a handful of others who believed in me. I may have felt alone in the crowd at that moment, but I knew that there was an army of people who helped propel me on this journey.

A voice came across the public-address system's speakers. It belonged to Roger Penske, chairman of the Indianapolis Motor Speedway. As a race-team owner, it was said that Penske "owned" the Speedway; his cars had won the 500 on 18 occasions prior to January of 2020, when he bought the historic facility from the Hulman-George family, its stewards since 1945. Now it was no longer said tongue-in-cheek; Roger really did own the place.

"Drivers," Penske instructed, "start your engines!"

Up and down the starting grid, 33 engines roared to life.

As sentimental as I was, it was time to focus. I climbed into the flagstand and put on the radio headset connecting me with the officials in the race-control suite.

"Pace car, move out!" the radio barked. I raised the yellow flag. I turned to Milo Ventimiglia and asked, "Any final questions?" But he was calm, at ease. I had the sense that, like me, it was not lost on him what an amazing opportunity he was getting, although his ceremonial duties would end after the initial start of the race.

"Starter and pace car," said a voice on the radio. "This is one to green." That meant that after this one final pace lap, the race would get underway. My nerves were now calm. They had to be. There was no room for doubt. Millions would be watching on the worldwide TV broadcast, and, more importantly, a mistake on my part could cost a driver and team a potential shot at millions of dollars. Or worse. But I knew what I was doing. I had been flagging races for 26 years.

Then again, this was the Indianapolis 500.

Had there been room in my head right now for stray thoughts, one would surely have been, "How in the world did an Aspie like me get here?"

It's true: At the age of 20, I had been diagnosed with Asperger syndrome, a condition on the autism spectrum. There were times before and after that diagnosis when I'd given up hope of working, hope of contributing to the world, hope of normal, everyday relationships; I'd given up hope, period.

Yet here I was, with the eyes of millions of fans, hundreds of team members, and 33 race drivers on me, watching my every move.

The race director's calm voice was now in my ear. "Starter, the field is in turn three, stand by … field is in four …"

Here, all traces of calm disappeared. His voice exploded—"GREEN, GREEN, GREEN!"—and my right arm waved furiously. The race was underway. This was all real.

It's Race Day in Indianapolis 1989

IT WAS MAY 28, 1989, AND OVER THE IMS SPEAKERS A VOICE I knew well was singing, "As I dream upon the moonlight on the Wabash…" I may have only been 6 years old, but already the pre-race ceremonies of the Indianapolis 500 were as sacred to me as a church service. I knew that Jim Nabors and "Back Home Again in Indiana" closed out the festivities, and that the race would be underway shortly. The skies were extra sunny and perfectly blue.

As the music faded, I turned to my dad. I wanted to ask a thousand questions about anything and everything related to the race, but I was so excited that I couldn't speak. Instead, I looked across the track to the infield and the places where my dad and I had been. The month of May in Indianapolis was literally a month-long affair in those days, and we lived not far from the track, so after school and on weekends he and I would watch practice and qualifying from the small infield bleachers. Today, I felt special; we were here for the race itself, my first 500, and I was in the actual grandstands, the largest expanse of seating anywhere in the world. The Speedway is massive, a 2.5-mile rectangle. Our seats were up high, between turns one and two.

"Gentlemen, start your engines!" This time, the command came from Mary F. Hulman, matriarch of the Hulman-George family and widow of Tony Hulman, the Indiana businessman who had rescued the track from potential ruin after it sat fallow and overgrown with weeds during World War II. I adjusted the ear protection I was wearing; I looked around and with youthful curiosity wondered why more people didn't wear something similar. I thought back to my first visit to the track, and what seemed like deafening noise. It was bad; I remember screaming loudly and trying to run away from my dad, but I wanted to be there even if the sound sliced through me like so many invisible knives. Today, I better understand my sensitivity to sound, but as a boy there was no way I could explain to my dad that it hurt me all the way to my toes. We discovered later that earplugs made it manageable.

The cars rolled past us for the first time. I had never seen the entire field of cars at once, 33 starters in 11 rows of three, and I was screaming in elation. My favorite driver, Al Unser, was in the middle of the front row, and I was hoping that he would win like he did in 1987. That was Al's fourth victory at Indy, making him only the second man, after A.J. Foyt, to win the 500 four times. I knew Al's fourth win very well; I had watched it endlessly on the VHS tape I had. The same was true with Rick Mears's third win, in 1988. I would watch and re-watch those races, and others. I may have been only 6, but I had watched the 500 more than many fans do in a lifetime.

As we watched the second of the field's three pace laps, the anticipation was crushing. In minutes, these cars and drivers would be hurtling past us at over 200 miles per hour. I kept yelling, "True colors!" That was a song featured in TV commercials for Kodak film; I was a sponge when it came to advertising slogans, but this one fit the moment because I was suddenly mesmerized by the colors that filled my vision. The paint liveries on the passing cars glistened in the sun; the bright clothing worn by the people in the infield looked like an image from a Kaleidoscope; atop each section of grandstands, flags blew in the breeze and displayed the colors—green, yellow, red, and more—of the flags the chief starter would be using. I had those flags memorized, and at school I made sure that everyone in my class knew what they meant.

When the field came by for the final time before the start, I looked up at one of the green flags waving above our section. That was the color, of course, that would signal the start of the race. At home, I had a souvenir checkered flag I had waved at a preschool Big Wheel rally and a kindergarten tricycle-and-bicycle day. Now I wished that I had a green flag to show everyone.

For several seconds, I was lost in the movements of that flag; I tended to fixate on things that flowed, spun, or waved. I was jolted back to consciousness by the revving of engines and the deep, booming voice of Tom Carnegie, the track's famed announcer. Both of those sounds told one and all that the race was underway.

No one forgets their first time seeing the start of the Indy 500. For me, it was a sensory explosion of sound, smell, and sight. I was still years away from being diagnosed with Asperger syndrome, and today I wonder: Had my condition been known, would my parents have ever brought me to the race? I'm glad they did; I was overstimulated but loved every moment.

I was too young to understand the nuances of racing. Things like fuel mileage, drafting, and tire wear were beyond me. I did know that Al Unser's car stopped coming around after just 68 of the race's 200 laps; his car had suffered a clutch failure. But his son, named Al Jr., was also in the race, so I had someone new to cheer for. On that day, there was an epic battle between Al Jr. and Brazilian driver Emerson Fittipaldi, who was described as a two-time Formula 1 World Champion. I didn't know what Formula 1 was, all I knew was Fittipaldi's red-and-white car needed to finish behind Al Jr.'s car, blue and white with red trim. As they passed our seats at the start of lap 199, with less than two full laps to go, Al Jr. was leading, but barely. Emerson was right on his tail. Even at 6, I understood the importance of the Indianapolis 500, and that any driver with a chance at victory would take it.

Fittipaldi took his chance entering turn three. He tried

an inside pass, and the two cars touched. Whether you chose to blame Emerson or Al Jr., the outcome was the same: Unser Jr. hit the wall, while Fittipaldi managed to keep his car rolling. The yellow flag waved for the crash, and Fittipaldi, running the final lap at a reduced caution speed, won the 1989 Indianapolis 500.

My memories of that day, oddly enough, do not include what it was like to arrive at the track, but our departure is still vivid in my memory. I was furious. First my hero, Al Unser, had fallen out of the event, and then his son had lost a thrilling race in a heartbreaking fashion. I cried in anger. But I also remember being astonished at the number of people leaving the track. I had read and heard everywhere that 400,000 "from all over the world" attended the race, but in the morning they arrived in waves, from dawn right up until race time. At day's end, it seemed like they all left at once, and I quickly gained an appreciation for how big a number 400,000 was.

I went to sleep that night, and many nights thereafter, feeling certain that I'd be a part of that event someday. There was no question about it: I would be a race driver, and Tom Carnegie would announce my name as winner of the Indianapolis 500.

It was as if nothing else mattered. There was just one goal. I had a mission, and if my brain encountered anything it deemed irrelevant to that mission, I had no time or patience for it. I was going to win that race one day.

I had no way of knowing that what I dreamed would be a straight road to that goal would instead be a long, circuitous route. Yes, it ended at the Indianapolis Motor Speedway, but rather than sitting low in a race car, I would see the 500 from a more elevated position.

—— A Defining, Prophetic Gift ——

THE INDY 500. IT WAS ALL I TALKED ABOUT WHEN I RETURNED to school in August. After experiencing what I felt was heaven on Earth, I didn't want to know anything else. I wore out at least one VCR that summer watching my collection of 500s, the four from 1986–1989. My interest was expanding, though. Instead of just cheering on the Unsers, I had grown increasingly intrigued by the flags I had seen. The ABC TV broadcast of the 1988 race included a report on race procedures, including the starts. They interviewed the 500's longtime chief steward, Tom Binford, who said that if the starting field looks nicely aligned as it rolls out of turn four, the folks in race control flip on the green lights that are spaced around the track while chief starter Duane Sweeney displays the green flag.

ABC showed camera views from above and behind Sweeney's shoulder. To a 6-year-old, those angles made the starter's stand look like a position unmatched in sports. I was awed that one person had a job with that much responsibility, and that Mr. Sweeney's motions with his flag were so clean, crisp, precise, and dynamic. With my little souvenir checkered flag, I imitated his style, but the flag was now falling apart, almost in tatters.

By summer's end, that souvenir flag was no longer in any shape to be waved. My dad took notice and one day he came home with a surprise for me: a full set of racing flags. I jumped, I screamed, and I immediately went to the green flag. I'd wanted one from the moment I watched the breeze rustling the green flag atop our grandstand section in May.

These flags were a bit smaller than an official set that would be used in the race, but they were perfect for my young hands. Besides, my dad said he bought them at the Indianapolis Motor Speedway Museum, so I treated them as if they were the real thing.

As summer closed out and the family VCR got a break during the day while I was at school, my flag-waving technique was being honed whenever possible. I made sure to watch as much televised racing as I could, both cheering on different drivers and watching the way various starters waved their flags. But nothing matched the drama of ABC's over-the-shoulder footage of Duane Sweeney, so lots of my non-school hours were devoted to re-watching those VHS 500s and conducting my own "flag along from home" sessions.

I'm not sure if my parents thought it peculiar that I spent so much time with my flags. Sure, most kids have some specific activity they'll enjoy, but I waved those flags hour after hour, repetition followed by more repetition. It never got old. Even on my umpteenth replay of a race, I was excited by every green and yellow flag. It meant another opportunity to mimic every motion and adjust it to fit my own form.

My dad told me we wouldn't be attending the race in 1990, because he had work commitments. He is a church pastor, so a commitment is a commitment. That was a hard blow, but he secretly went to great lengths to make it up to me. A member of his church, a lady named JoAnn, worked at the United States Auto Club, the organization that sanctioned and officiated the Indianapolis 500. He asked if she thought it might be possible for her to get Duane Sweeney's autograph.

Sometime later he got a phone call from JoAnn, and he said later that the flag was the last thing on his mind because she sounded like she was in serious physical distress. He knew that she suffered from severe emphysema and remembers her out of breath, saying, "Pastor, get over here quick!" He was sure this was an emergency, and broke a few traffic laws on his way to her house. Her front door was open. He rushed in and found her seated in the kitchen.

My dad was a bit confused and asked, "What's wrong?"

"Oh, nothing," said JoAnn. "If I sounded out of breath, it's because I had just walked out to get the paper."

Then she stood up and said, "I've got something for you." She left the room and brought back two signed photos of Duane Sweeney. Unfortunately, they were made out to "Erin" rather than "Aaron." But any concerns on my dad's part disappeared when she said, "Oh, there's one more thing…"

This "one more thing" ended up becoming something of a beacon in my life. JoAnn produced a checkered flag; it was one of Duane Sweeney's checkered flags, one he had meant to use in the 500 just a few months later.

It's an Indy 500 tradition that before the event, all 33 qualified drivers sign two checkered flags. At the end of the race, the starter waves them both over the winner in a unique double-checkered flourish. Then one flag goes to the winner, and the Speedway museum gets the other. Every year, Duane's wife made those two flags by hand, and the one I got was originally destined to be one of those two flags used on race day.

When my dad learned of this, he was surprised enough to ask JoAnn how and why she ended up with this special gift from Duane … for *me*.

She said, "I called Duane and told him that he had a big fan here in town, and he felt it was right to send one of these flags to a true fan. His wife has severe arthritis, and she told him she wasn't making another flag. But he responded by saying that he doesn't have many fans, so she'd *have* to make him another flag for the race."

My dad came home and proved that, much like JoAnn, he had a flair for the dramatic. He gave me the signed pictures and then left the room to grab "one more thing." There's a photo of the moment he handed me that flag, and I think I had a bigger natural smile than you'll find in any other photo from my childhood.

By this point, I was 7 years old, so I'm sure I didn't fully appreciate the true uniqueness of this gift. Could anyone at that age grasp that this was a handmade item, one of a kind, and could never be replaced? That I was given something reserved only for winners of the 500? But I did know this: I could now wave a checkered flag exactly like the one Duane Sweeney waved.

We've all heard the cliché that important events can send ripples through our lives, much like a pebble dropped into a pond. With that flag, it was as if someone tossed a bowling ball from the roof of a house into a kiddie pool. The splash was big, and my passion for motorsports grew and expanded, as waves do. More than ever, racing was everything to me. Nothing else mattered.

The Quest for Silverstone

"WHAT DO YOU WANT TO BE WHEN YOU GROW UP?" ASKED my kindergarten teacher.

"Race car driver," I replied.

"What do you want to be when you grow up?" asked my first-grade teacher.

"Race car driver."

Same question every year, same answer every year. I'm sure my teachers didn't understand me.

Academically, most things came easy to me. There were, however, mysterious things like prepositional phrases that teetered on the impossible. It's odd that I'm a published writer, because writing was not something I did in school. Actually, I didn't do much. I talked about the weather, mostly because I was terrified of severe weather; an ominous forecast left me paralyzed with fear. If there was a chance of a violent storm, I did all I could to be sure I wasn't in school.

Missing school was commonplace for me. It simply wasn't something I felt was important when I was in, say, the second grade. Why would I? What could I possibly learn in class that would have any relevance to what goes on in a race car? In hindsight, my strength and determination in setting and pursuing goals was a big detriment to my education.

To say I was uncomfortable in school would be doing a disservice to the idea of comfort. I tried to socialize with classmates, but I lacked the ability to talk about anything but racing and the weather. Oh, and I also had a fear of nuclear war with the Soviet Union; again, I could talk about that because I was afraid of it. As early as kindergarten, I talked to another student about atomic bombs, and that went as well as you might imagine. The other kid ran away, not fully understanding what I was talking about but having a newfound fear of mushrooms.

Day in and day out, I was lonely, the quintessential unmotivated student. When I did take interest in something, it often turned into a negative. For example, games sparked my interest, and my abnormally fast reflexes, combined with my ability to harness the power of rote memorization, gave me an advantage.

Two subjects I enjoyed were math and state capitals. In my first- and second-grade classes, we'd play a fast-paced game where two students would go head-to-head and the winning student moved on to the next desk and the next opponent. Typically, the game ended with no one seated where they'd been when the game started, because each student won some and lost some. It didn't happen that way when I played. I could go an entire session undefeated, so I kept moving while everyone else remained in place. As a result, I was probably the only one having any fun. To make it easier on the other students, I was either banned or allowed to play just one question before I was named the "retired champion." This hurt me all the way down to the plasma in my blood. I finally enjoyed being a part of something, and now I was banned or "retired." What was I supposed to do, throw the games? I was just a kid.

"Alone in a crowd." So many people with Asperger's explain their lives this way, and this is how I would define my school years. Those fleeting moments taking part in a game with the group were powerful, yet rare. My first-grade teacher overlooked me, but my second-grade teacher, Mrs. Jendra, made sure to find a way of keeping me engaged in the activities.

In the past, as soon as I was "retired" from games, I was given busy work. Mrs. Jendra instead gave me a "promotion" and allowed me to lead the game, reading the questions or holding the flashcards. This was the first time I felt comfortable in a social setting of any kind. Even in second grade, I thought it strange that I couldn't read in front of a class, and that having a conversation with more than one person was so overwhelming that soon I could not speak, yet being the "host" of the game felt natural. Mrs. Jendra noticed that, as well.

She did everything right, even before we understood what "right" was. She used tricks not yet identified to make sure I was engaged. She allowed me to go on tangents about racing, knowing that she could probably then redirect my energy to the work at hand. I may still have been alone in a crowded cafeteria, but there was a newfound feeling of being *worth* something. She couldn't help me crack the code of the prepositional phrase, but I learned the need-to-know stuff of second grade. But her lasting legacy occurred in the closing weeks of the school year.

Think back on your own school days. Did you ever have a teacher ask a question or utter a statement so profound yet so simple that it shattered your view of the world? I hope you can say yes, and I hope that everyone can point to a teacher who helped change the trajectory of their lives. Perhaps this is most common at the high-school or college level, but for me it happened in second grade.

As one of my racing monologues unfolded on this day, Mrs. Jendra flipped the conversation. She said, "Okay, Aaron, you've mentioned Formula 1 several times. Tell me, where does Formula 1 race in England?"

I proudly responded, "Silverstone." But she knew of my capacity for rote memorization, so she immediately asked, "Where is Silverstone?"

That threw me off for a bit; I thought it was a trick. In a questioning tone, I replied, "England?"

"Okay," she said. "And where is England?"

Wow. I knew it was a name that went with Silverstone, but I had no idea that it was a country, or where it was located. Just like that, I instantly became interested in the places where races occurred.

It was a shame that her question about Silverstone came at the end of a school year, because suddenly my world no longer ended at the barriers that surrounded race tracks. That very day, I started browsing through the encyclopedias at home, something I never had done because they contained no information on racing. Because of my deep interest in racing, I was learning about things *outside* of racing. I was curious not only about these places, but about what life was like for those who lived in these places.

I'm not sure how my life would have gone had this passion not been created that day. Mrs. Jendra identified my interest, and then stepped into *my* world to show me there was something beyond that small world. For the first time, I realized that there was more to life, and more to racing, than *just* racing.

The Story of Third Grade and Four Small Sagas of Kickball, Eye Contact, Learning that Right Can be Wrong, and a Rock

THIS IS A BOOK ABOUT A JOURNEY TO A DREAM, AND NO journey is complete without drama. Much of the drama in my early life involved the struggle to avoid school. I'm often asked if I was bullied in school. If I was, I would have probably been oblivious to it because I was too busy explaining to my teachers my obsession with racing.

Recess was an awkward time for me because instead of talking to a teacher inside, I was now talking outside. My first-grade teacher once gave me an ultimatum, "If you talk to me about racing one more time, you're never going to recess again!" Mrs. Jendra in second grade made no such threat, but did her best to expand the topics I was interested in. My third-grade teacher? Well …

Shortly into the school year, she gave me the, "You're not talking to me" dissertation. Adding to my struggles at recess was that my family had moved from the west side of Indy to the north side, so this was a new school for me. I didn't know anyone.

I tried to partake in America's schoolyard pastime, kickball, but there was one big problem with that: I found out that it isn't so much a sport as it is a starting point for future politicians. Why? Because it isn't a sport, but rather one long debate after another. No one in our games could agree on whether a base runner was safe or out. Every call, even something as basic as catching a fly ball, was subject to interpretation. For a person like me who knew the rules, this was another infuriating aspect of life that just shouldn't have been the way it was.

So I fixed it.

After a couple of mind-numbing weeks of listening to these debates, I stepped in to become the adjudicator of kickball justice and named myself commissioner of our playground kickball league. No one objected, and I finally had a calling at recess. Working first base and keeping the game moving was something I was proud of.

While the recess problem had been solved it was a long school year indoors. Again, this was long before Asperger's was a recognized diagnosis and society was more rigid on social rules. For many of us on the spectrum, it takes just a wee bit of frustration to make *everything* not work, and my third-grade teacher gave me many things to be frustrated about. I simply did not know how to adjust to her ways. I was too young to use a word like "paranoia" at this point in my life, but I had the feeling that she was out to get me in any way she could. And halfway through the school year, she found her ultimate weapon.

Direct eye contact is something I have always struggled with. Whenever I approached her desk to drop off a paper or ask a question, I'd always look over her shoulder or above her. She always counteracted this with a stern, "Look at me when I talk to you!"

I'd comply and attempt to deal with the very real physical discomfort that came with her glares. If I had to ask her something, my heart would pound. Beat after beat. I feared the journey to her desk and the inevitable reprimand for my lack of eye contact. Sometimes when I averted my eyes, she would threaten to write my name on the blackboard, which happened to students who misbehaved. To me, that punishment was the equivalent of a 25-to-life prison sentence, something I knew I'd never rebound from. It was almost as if she was looking for a way to make this happen. And one day, she got her wish.

In her classroom, the seating arrangement changed every two weeks. There was no such thing as getting comfortable, because just as I was getting used to where everyone was now—not an easy process for me—we would all change seats again. And it was not just a matter of taking different seats; even the *arrangement* of the seats would change. Chairs might be arranged in a five-by-five grid, or in small squares of four, or in a pentagon configuration.

In one version, we were in a giant square and the students to my left and right were the class clowns. Now, clowning was fine when it didn't involve me. I had no time for it; all my energy was spent getting my work done, to be sure I didn't end up with homework.

One secret I kept from everyone was the sheer exhaustion a school day gave me. There were so many struggles, things I just didn't understand, and I thought everyone must have been stronger than me. For example, I had a fear of fire drills. The fire alarm caused a genuine pain response in my body; imagine being stabbed in the arms and legs with thousands of small needles, and you'll have a rough sense of what it was like for me.

The exhaustion came from *processing* all of the things a school day presented. It took so much effort just to hear the lessons, because I couldn't filter out the ambient noise, the typical classroom sounds, the whispers, or, in this case, the clowning.

It happened during a social-studies class. Ever since my second-grade teacher had unlocked my curiosity about the world I was a sponge on anything related to new places. On this day, we were learning to read maps. Now, I was already familiar with the road atlas; on family trips to Nebraska, I would pass the long drive studying the lines on the map and the highways they represented. The map we were learning in class was different, though, and I was excited. But the students on either side of me, the two class clowns, were obviously bored; they thought it would be fun to throw a pencil back and forth over my desk.

Up went the pencil, down went the pencil. Up went the pencil, down went the pencil. Up, down …

I was getting mad, but I didn't say anything. I never allowed myself to speak out on things like this. My goal was a supreme level of stoicism. Anything else might result in a conversation with the teacher, and that would require eye contact.

Up, down. The teacher had to be silently condoning this attempt at a new Olympic event, the pencil toss, because the alternative was that she was completely blind to what was going on in her classroom.

Up, down … and a near-interception by Aaron Likens! But at least there was a deflection, and an interruption of their silly game.

Totally out of character, and slamming my desk for emphasis, I yelled, "Would you *please* stop throwing the pencil!"

The room froze. The kid to my right said, "Oh, why didn't you say something?" I looked blankly at him; I was confused. How did he not *know* they were bothering me? This may have been my first experience with the "theory of mind" idea that says, "I *think*, therefore you should *know*." But this was no time to discuss what he knew or didn't know. The teacher was highly angry with this fracas in her classroom. There was no thought given to who played what role in this disturbance; the class clowns and I were all told to write our names on the blackboard.

What was going on? This was the end for me, I was sure of it. I pleaded my case, and all I got in return was the threat of more name-writing. I'd done nothing wrong, and I was sure she knew that, yet I was clumped in with the clowns. I lost any respect I still had for the teacher. This did not change my daily demeanor. I remained stoic, but it all added to the exhaustion I felt.

I needed an outlet from the pressure of school and did my best to be busy when I got home each day. If the Nintendo games weren't cutting it, I would tear around the neighborhood on my bicycle. But I had a horrible streak of getting gnats in my eyes, and my eyes were sensitive anyway, so I parked the bike. What was I to do? I had so much rage building from misunderstandings, eye contact, and the idea that this teacher had doled out the classroom version of vigilante justice for no reason other than "just because." Then, just when I needed something good to happen, I found my very own flagstand.

It was a large rock that sat at the entrance of our cul-de-sac. It stood about a foot high and was the perfect roadside spot to stand on and wave a checkered flag at whatever cars drove by. This road wasn't busy, so I might stand there for 30 minutes and see no cars, but that was okay. Once I took to the rock with my Duane Sweeney checkered flag, the same flag that would have waved over the Indianapolis Motor Speedway saw regular action flying over the corner of Ripon Court and Fordham Avenue.

It was an amazing feeling. Each time a car came my way, I would emulate the style Duane used during Indy 500 qualifications, ending each driver's time-trial run with a grand wave of the checkered flag. In return, I'd get honks, smiles, and waves. It wasn't hard to imagine that instead of Ford Tempos and Geo Metros rolling slowly past me, these were the fast cars of legends like Foyt, Mears, or the Unsers.

The fact that I had to get to my rock flagstand every afternoon gave me further motivation to avoid having any homework. I started to develop my own style of flag-waving. As I worked through all of this, it was not out of the ordinary for me to spend hours each day on that rock. Once again, I had no idea what my parents thought; I don't know if they were concerned at all with this admittedly odd hobby. But as strange as it may have been, it was the outlet I needed.

All the sagas of third grade were necessary and important lessons that would help me to handle things that would happen later on in life.

Thoughts and Reflections on the Rock in 1992

WHEN THE SCHOOL YEAR CAME TO A MERCIFUL END, THE summer flew by. Before I knew it, I was headed back to school. It was never far from my mind anyway because the school building was only a block and a half from my house.

The first day of school was like sticking my hand into a covered basket with a sign that warned, "BEWARE! Angry spiders inside!" Odds are there are none, so the end result was going to be better than what I feared. But this wasn't always the case; in first grade, the stress led me to throw up all over my desk. Imagine having that be your first impression for 25 other kids! The person who first observed that "first impressions are the most important" had no idea just how crippling they can be for a person on the spectrum. And since I went through that on my *first* first day, I knew it was going to happen again.

That's another cornerstone of my life as an Aspie: Whatever happens first *always* has to happen.

Every year, I tried to get out of going to school on the first day. I thought I was a superb actor, and if there were categories at the Oscars for Best Headache, Best Sore Throat, and Best Stomach Ache, I'd have won them all. But my dad, knowing me so well, reached the point where he no longer believed any performance I gave. So I went, and there was no opening-day disaster as fourth grade began. Actually, the first day was kind of amazing.

Mrs. Colvin, the teacher, was extremely welcoming. Gone was the mandatory eye contact and the threats over me speaking too much about certain subjects. In their place was another teacher who, like Mrs. Jendra, utilized my strengths to get me interested in my weaknesses.

As good as I had always been with numbers, I had no interest in learning division, a key feature of fourth-grade math. To get me motivated, Mrs. Colvin said, "Aaron, if the winner of the Indy 500 averaged one mile per hour, how long would it take them to go 500 miles? And after you have that answer, do the same distance at 1.5 miles per hour, and then go all the way up to 200." Her motivation was even more effective than she'd hoped, because now in all my classes—English, social studies, it didn't matter—I was using math to crack the code of average speeds.

Mrs. Colvin also didn't lay down rules on what I could or couldn't speak to her about during recess. This was a grand change of pace, but unless something odd happened in a race or there was a major weather event, I was happier to continue my reign as kickball commissioner. I'd been in this school for a year now, so I was no longer the new kid, and I was expected to take my post. The playground debates were long gone, and the games were fun.

There was one student who was a phenom when it came to kicking. Anytime he was at the plate, the fielders shifted backward, and still there was a risk of a home run. He kicked farther than anyone, and the way he transferred his energy to the ball was something to see.

He played every day. Remember, whatever happens first *always* has to happen, and the longer it goes on, the more impossible a change of course becomes. But there was a change one day in the spring of 1992, when he didn't come to the kickball lot. I knew he was in school, because I saw him in the hall. I couldn't help but wonder what was going on. Was something wrong? For once in my life, I decided to risk it; I left the field and went to find him, thinking about what I might say if we struck up a conversation.

He was standing by the school doors, looking down as if he had been crushed by someone or something. When I got close to him, he looked up at me, sighed, and simply said, "My dog died this morning." That wasn't what I was expecting to hear, so I went ahead with the conversation I had scripted in my mind.

I said, "Oh, okay. Um, do you want to go play kickball now?"

He did not reply. He looked even more defeated than he had when I walked up. I went back to the kickball lot and umpired the game, at the same time wondering about his cold response.

As I walked home after school, the gears were turning in my head. There were several things I was working on: How did others know what to say and when to say it with more ease than me? Why did it take me longer to talk than others? And finally, what was with that guy's non-response to my kickball question?

I had no answers, so I took to my refuge, my rock flag-stand, to think about things.

I started waving my flag, but I got more upset with every car that passed. That boy had no reason to be mad at me. I mean, he was in school, and he wasn't busy, but he didn't want to play kickball, apparently because his dog had died …

Wait. Wait! His dog had *died*. I had a dog, Missy the Maltese, and in a story for the school paper I wrote that she would "always be by my side, because she's the best dog in the world." What if this other kid had thought *his* dog was the best in the world? *Argh …*

How had I not picked up on his sadness? I was flooded with an emotion I had not experienced: empathy. It overwhelmed me. I stepped off my rock and went home, not feeling well. I was angry at myself, to a level that was un-rivaled to that point. It had taken me almost five hours of thinking about that social interaction to realize what happened. That bothered me.

A couple of things happened the next day. The first was that I *almost* apologized, but I didn't. Apologies are always awkward, so I tend to avoid them even when they're needed. Secondly, I became more fearful than ever about speaking if I didn't have to. I had said the absolute worst thing at the absolute wrong time, suggesting a kickball game after this kid had lost his pet, and I didn't want to risk doing that again.

I still think of that episode when I'm unsure about how to interact with someone.

For a while, I made myself scarce at the kickball field. Instead, I talked with the teacher about the weather and racing. If I stuck with things I understood, I wouldn't be risking another bad incident.

Soon enough, it was the end of my fourth-grade school year. That made me sad. I knew I might never have another teacher like Mrs. Colvin.

I think about Mrs. Jendra and Mrs. Colvin frequently, and it makes me sad to think that they don't know how my story turned out. A teacher can change a child's life, planting the seeds that lead to him or her fulfilling their potential … and yet their last image of that child may be of them leaving the classroom on that last day because school is out for the summer.

Those teachers won't know the number of students who look back and wish they had managed to stop and say, in the most solemn of voices, "Thank you for what you've done for me. Thank you for believing in me. And most of all, thank you for not just teaching me, but reaching me."

A Cold Day in May

I NEVER FIGURED OUT HOW MY DAD SCORED THE TICKETS, but in 1992 he and I went to my second Indianapolis 500. We sure picked a great year. Our seats seemed like the best in the house, in the paddock penthouse section, above and behind the start/finish line. My dad complained—jokingly, I think—that we wouldn't see the turns. But for me, the seats were perfect. I could see Duane Sweeney perform in person, just in front of me, while also daydreaming that I'd be driving the first car to take his double checkered flags.

It was blustery and unseasonably cold for the 500 that year. It also took us an eternity to get to the track on race morning. With traffic moving so slowly, there was plenty of time to observe others among the hundreds of thousands descending upon the track. One incident that sticks with me: A man driving a car with Ohio plates put his car in park, jumped out, and loudly asked his passenger, "Do you have the tickets?" The passenger must have said no, and the driver began thrashing about in the trunk of his car. As we passed him, he yelled to the heavens, "They're on the kitchen table at home!" Oops!

When we finally got to the track and reached our seats, we found the wind was blowing in our faces. The wind-chill temperature that morning was 28 degrees. I was 9 years old, and if we'd been anywhere else, I'd have done everything I could to leave and get to someplace warm. But this was the Indianapolis Motor Speedway, so the weather was not a concern to me. But I almost had to remind myself to breathe as pre-race ceremonies began; the place, the race, and its traditions meant so much to me. They call the 500 the Greatest Spectacle in Racing, and to me there is no doubt.

Under the dreariest of gray skies, the field rolled off for the parade laps. Unlike the shimmering colors of 1989, today's view was more like I imagined Siberia looks just before a blizzard. As if in response to the gloom, polesitter Roberto Guerrero crashed on the backstretch during one of the parade laps, and French rookie Philippe Gache spun moments later in turn four. Cold tires were blamed; the rubber was not generating enough heat on the slow parade laps to make good traction.

With my dad still grumbling about our view, the field got ready for the start, a moment that produces hope, fear, and a little prayer. It was my first time seeing the beginning of the race from the frontstretch, but I don't remember much. It's a strange thing, to see and feel that explosion of sound and motion but not be able to replay it in your mind; maybe your brain takes it all in, but it's too big to store as a memory. Was I watching the 33 cars? Was I watching Duane Sweeney? I believe I was watching both, but I'm not sure.

The 500 itself resembled a county-fair demolition derby. Many drivers later complained that cold tires and gusting winds made for unpredictable handling. Too often, Sweeney had to reach for his yellow flags. Even the most experienced drivers had trouble; Mario Andretti, Rick Mears, Tom Sneva, Emerson Fittipaldi, and Arie Luyendyk were past Indy 500 winners, but all of them were eliminated after crashing in 1992. It was a brutal race, and several drivers suffered injuries. Any time a human being is strapped into a car traveling well over 200 MPH, the risk of serious harm is there.

Nearing the finish, Michael Andretti, Mario's son, looked like he was in control. He had led 160 laps. Now, with just 11 laps to go and a 30-second lead, track announcer Tom Carnegie used four words he had often used when referring to unlucky Mario: "Andretti is slowing down." He was out of the race with a fuel-pressure issue.

The race turned instantly from a runaway to a fantastic two-car duel between Al Unser Jr. and Scott Goodyear. Just three years earlier, on my first race day at the track, Unser Jr. was just over a lap away from a win before the contact with

Fittipaldi. That was in my mind. But my favorite driver—Al Jr. had taken that role from his dad—had gone from running a distant second to leading the race.

In the last 10 laps, Goodyear crept closer and closer to the tail of Al Jr.'s car. The crowd's cheering went up a dozen decibels each lap. It was thrilling.

I had waited the entire race to watch Duane Sweeney wave the white flag and then the twin checkered flags, but when the two lead cars took the white, they were running so closely that I could not take my eyes off of them. I missed the white flag. I held my breath for the next 40-plus seconds, looking toward turn four, until they came back into view. Al Jr. was still leading, but Goodyear was gaining on him. Goodyear made a last-minute attempt to pass as they neared the famous "yard of bricks" that serves as the start/finish line at the Speedway, but Al Jr. held him back, winning by 0.043 seconds. It was the closest margin of victory in Indianapolis 500 history. It had been so tight that I screamed at my dad, "Who won? Who won?" When he told me, I couldn't believe it.

I guess I missed the checkered flags, too.

Walking back to our van, I skipped along, floating on air. I had never been happier. My favorite driver had won, I got to see my favorite starter wave his flags, and it all happened with my dad right beside me.

I'm not sure exactly when I said it, but at some point after the race I said to my dad, "Those seats weren't bad after all, were they?"

Finding My Way Before Moving into Another World

AS FIFTH GRADE BEGAN, SO DID THE USUAL CLASSROOM dynamics. My teacher was young, and once again, I was banned from classroom games but allowed to "host" or do some advanced math problems.

Away from school, there was a segment on the local news about a small track at the Indiana State Fairgrounds where kids raced tiny cars called Quarter Midgets. I told my dad, and he made a few calls. He spoke with Tony George, president of the Indianapolis Motor Speedway, about the steps to get into that type of racing. It was very expensive, so money was going to be an obstacle, but there was a chance that we could get some sponsorship from Jonathan Byrd, who owned a popular cafeteria and was a longtime IndyCar team owner and sponsor. My dad had done some work for Mr. Byrd, so as winter turned to spring in 1994, it looked like I might be on my way to fulfilling my destiny as the next great American racing champion of the universe.

But in October, my dad took a job in St. Louis. I had only remembered moving once, from one Indianapolis neighborhood to another, so this relocation was traumatic. Change is extremely tough for people with Asperger syndrome and other autism-spectrum disorders. It's said that moving is among the most stressful events in *anyone's* life; throw autism into the mix, and it becomes all the more upsetting.

The countdown to the first week of December and moving day was scary. I knew little about St. Louis, other than it had the Gateway Arch and a baseball team. I'd never heard of St. Louis having any connection to motorsports, so I figured this move was the end of my racing dream.

On my last day of school in Indianapolis, my dad had to

come and pick me up earlier than we planned. I was just too emotional. I only had one real friend in my class, but the idea of losing everyone and everything was overwhelming. It didn't help that I was given a "College Park Elementary School" pencil to remember them all by. I cried from the school to my house, and then until I went to sleep.

As the sun rose, it was time to move on, literally, toward our new home. The trip itself seemed like a bad omen: one of my cats had a severe accident in the crate, and then, 50 miles down the road, my mom's car caught fire. This was all before cell phones, and when we got to a gas station to call AAA, our dog broke free and my mom had to make a diving stop to keep her from running into the road. It was a misadventure in moving, and I worried that this 260-mile move would put me in a world I knew nothing about.

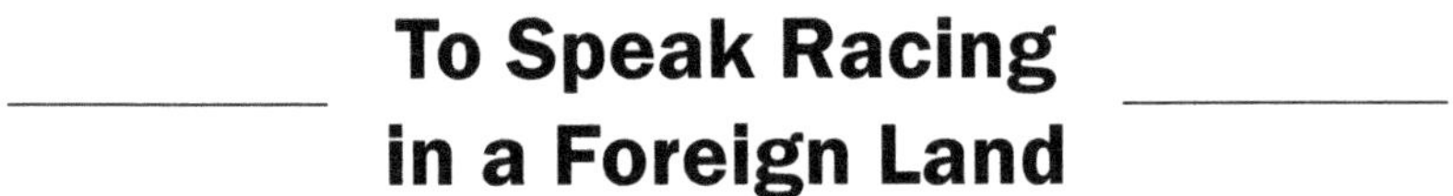

To Speak Racing in a Foreign Land

THOSE OF US ON THE AUTISM SPECTRUM LOVE TALKING about "our Kansas." My first book, "Finding Kansas," took its title from this idea, which goes like this: If you only felt normal and could only function socially within the borders of Kansas, where would you want to live? The answer would obviously be Kansas.

For me, Kansas was racing. Well, sometimes the weather, but mostly racing. In Indianapolis, people at least knew what I was talking about when I mentioned the Speedway or the 500. In St. Louis, it was another story.

I've mentioned being alone in a crowd, but now I was

alone *outside* the crowd. My efforts at talking about weather or racing were, for the most part, ignored, and I was confused. I kept trying, but no matter what I did, I was on the outside looking in.

My social awkwardness and unintentional aloofness didn't help. My early school days in St. Louis were a never-ending cavalcade of embarrassing blowups. For instance, gym class was a non-stop showcase of my ineptitude. One day, we were playing hockey—a game I knew very little about—and I was assigned to be a "defender." Hockey was big in St. Louis; they had the NHL Blues, with the great Brett Hull. Everyone knew hockey, but I didn't.

Being a defender, of course, meant that I had to defend. I had to get in the way, or use the stick to get the ball from the other team, so when my team had possession, I stayed back by the goal. My team kept yelling at me to attack, but I didn't; I had been told that I was a defender, and my mind insisted that I follow rules and directions. The PE teacher seemed to revel in watching the train wreck I was, because he offered no pointers on how to play the role of defender.

Our mid-year move meant that my fifth-grade time was only one semester. I tried using whatever social skills I had to engage other students in conversation, but they were having none of it. Instead of Unser and Mears, they talked about Ozzie Smith and Willie McGee, and I didn't know those people. I was dying on the inside. Depression was setting in.

The summer of '94 didn't do much to cheer things up. I attempted to socialize with the neighborhood kids, but that went poorly. The only bright spot came when I organized a bicycle race and got to use my flags.

Adjusting to this new world on the Mississippi River wasn't going well. As sixth grade began, the social divide I felt somehow grew even wider. Attending school was becoming a truly painful experience; the teacher's methods were not clicking with me, the other students grew tired of my inability to grasp their sports, and I was left wondering at the end of each day how other kids could move about with such grace and ease when it came to socializing.

Nothing about this was enjoyable, so missing school became the norm. I would simply refuse to go, and I used every trick in the book to achieve this. I doubt many people would blame me if they knew the pain I felt each day.

By the midpoint of sixth grade, I had missed more days than I had attended. I pushed my parents to look into homeschooling; I was alone in school, so why not be alone in a class at home and have a chance to learn without all of the other pressures? Thankfully, my parents agreed to give homeschooling a shot.

Oddly, on my last day of public school with my classmates, I grew sad again, much like I'd done in Indianapolis a year prior. But there was no celebration this time, no pencil to remember them by. As fast as I had arrived, I unceremoniously disappeared from their lives. However, I'm sure any time they watch hockey, they can't help but think of the kid whose name they can't remember but who made a mockery out of the position of defender.

I didn't know it at the time, but my life was about to change. Racing, the sport I longed to be a part of, was about to become a reality for me, and this is where my story truly begins.

The Pace Laps

IN THE DEAD OF A COLD WINTER'S NIGHT, A WOULD-BE burglar changed my life by breaking into our garage and stealing my dad's table saw. I knew nothing of this until my dad asked if I wanted to try racing go-karts. Of course I did, but I knew money was tight. He told me that instead of replacing this stolen saw, we could get a go-kart.

The drive to the kart shop, Trackside Motorsports, is still fresh in my memory. Each mile on the drive west of town seemed like a lifetime, and I kept waiting to wake up and find out that this was all a dream. But then we parked by the shop's door, exited the van, and walked in.

It was overwhelming to step into the shop. The mixed aroma of tires, oil, plastics, and new race suits must have been what heaven smelled like, and throughout the shop were beautiful karts. Some were basic, others anything but; I knew this was where a career began.

The shop owner talked to me about how a kart operates: gas on the right, brake on the left. I got a bit frustrated because I already knew such basic things. I kept asking what the track looked like, and she finally got out a diagram. I stared at it, visualizing racing lines and passing zones. I was only 12, but I was trying to savor the moment. This was destiny coming true!

When we left the shop without a kart, I was in disbelief. My dad assured me that I would be racing, and that the kart shop was waiting for a chassis someone was trading in. Sure enough, a couple of weeks later we brought home a chassis tied to the top of my dad's van. It was mine!

When we got home, my dad brought the kart into the living room. Sitting in it felt like the most exhilarating thing I had ever done. But there was a problem; we had no engine. Then, just like the wait for the chassis, a week or two went by and we got an engine.

My dad worked many nights in the garage prepping the kart. I didn't participate because I was useless when it came to tools. Even screwdrivers were beyond my skill set. Also, whenever I got any grease or oil on my hands, I'd rush inside to wash them. But I never once paused to think that maybe I was not cut out for this. I knew I would fly when I got behind the wheel.

Before my first time on an actual track, my dad thought it best that I get acclimated to the kart in a controlled environment. On a chilly weekend morning in early spring, we loaded the kart into the van and drove to his place of employment, where the parking lot was empty. My dad added the fuel, checked the oil and the tire pressure, and then it was time.

This was a parking lot. There were no lane markers, so I didn't know which way to go. Before the engine fired, my dad said, "Go around that light pole and then this light pole." I asked how we would know if I were fast? There was no finish line, no stopwatch. He told me to just get used to accelerating and braking, but I was trying to fly before I learned how to walk.

The suit was zipped up, the helmet fastened, and I lowered into the seat. After my dad started the engine, I played with the pedals, and was shocked at how responsive the throttle was.

Some markings on the parking lot made it easy to imagine a track, so after one slow lap I went full blast. When I tried to make one of my imaginary turns, I realized I was going way too fast, so I applied full brakes. That locked up the kart's rear axle, and I went into a nice 180-degree spin. I was afraid my dad would be angry that I spun, but he just restarted the engine and sent me back out. I reminded myself not to put every ounce of leg strength into braking.

I could only go around this parking lot so many times. I wanted the real thing, and when my dad was convinced that

I wouldn't be a danger on a real track, we went home and started making plans. In just seven days, I would arrive at the Widman County Park track to start what was sure to be a tale of extreme success.

—————— The First Green Flag ——————

THE DAYS LEADING UP TO THE FIRST OFFICIAL PRACTICE seemed longer than my 12 years on Earth. Not only this, but I kept remembering something the kart-shop owners said: that we should closely watch the weather, because Widman County Park was on land that was routinely flooded by the Meramec River in the spring. He said that two years earlier, in the flood of 1993, the St. Louis Karting Association couldn't run a single event at the track, and almost disbanded because of it. I feared this might happen again in '95, but the week leading to opening day was dry. When Saturday came, my dad woke me up at 6:00 a.m., and I got ready with no hesitation.

We started what became a tradition for us: stopping at the St. Louis Hills Donut Shop just as daylight arrived. Fueled by donuts and milk, it was time to see what I could do on a real track.

Ten turns packed into .35 miles. That's the sight that greeted me as we turned off Telegraph Road and I stared out at the field where the track sat. Just the sight of it shrouded in a slight fog and the crisp spring air was enough to ramp up my nerves.

For the first time in my life, I considered the dangers of going racing. I had seen crashes on television where the driver had been injured, but it never occurred to me that this could happen to *me*. To make matters worse, the waivers we signed at the gate read, in part, "By signing, you acknowledge that the event may cause injury or death …" This was risky. The document said so.

Fear and doubt crept in. Maybe I didn't want this after all. Perhaps I could have as much fun just watching others race. But even as a kid, I thought that my dad had done too much for me to turn back. Besides, crashes happened to *other* people. I'd be better and avoid it.

At 9:00 a.m., the track opened for practice. I'd like to tell you that right away I set a blistering pace, but that would be a lie. The rebuilt engine had to be broken in, which involved running a number of laps at quarter-speed and then half-speed. My dad explained it in technical terms, but what I heard was, "Go too fast, engine goes boom. No money to fix engine."

This was strange: Go out onto a track with no speed limit but be sure to limit your speed. Other karts kept passing me, and some of the adult drivers went by me at frightening speeds. I felt like I was riding a tricycle on an Interstate highway, with trucks blowing past me.

I had no idea, obviously, what full speed felt like. I just hoped the engine didn't go boom. Thankfully, it did not, and after the proper number of break-in laps, my dad waved me into the pits so we could change the oil.

At home, my dad changed the oil, and this time he said it was my turn; I'm sure he just wanted me to learn. I went along happily and took the funnel and then pulled the drain plug. That's when I remembered that I hated having oil or grease on my hands. I'm not sure what I did wrong, but my hand was quickly covered with the dirty, gritty oil, and I dropped the funnel with a shriek. My dad quickly stepped in, but I stood there in horror, running my fingers together and looking at the murky brown substance. My dad told me to grab a towel from the back of the van, and getting the oil off my hands was a huge relief.

So, this was racing. Thoughts of dealing with dirty oil on my hands had already replaced the fear of crashes and injury. Does *everything* have to be difficult?

Soon enough, I was back on track, and for me this session would be at speed. Full speed. I didn't have to worry about hurting the engine and ending my career before it had begun. I could focus on speed and finding the proper lines in the turns. And as I was doing that, I found myself encountering slower karts; time to learn how to pass!

I was shouting in my helmet: "To the left! To the right! Whoa! I out braked that guy!"

In stick-and-ball school sports, I had no athletic ability and was extremely awkward, physically uncoordinated. Behind the wheel, I felt like I had the precision of a surgeon. With each session, my confidence grew, except when I got behind one particular kart, #24.

I knew #24 was also on track for the first time, and his speed was slow. His favorite driver was Jeff Gordon, but Jeff Gordon he was not. I still can't figure out the problem I had with him; everyone else got around him quickly, but no matter what I did, I caught him in the wrong spot and had to back off. Then it would take several laps to get my speed back and start looking again for a place to overtake him. This ate up time and fuel and shortened my temper.

It was the last session of the day. I wanted to set a time that was close to the top two drivers; one was Jeremy Schrader, nephew to NASCAR driver Ken Schrader, and the other was Matt Krechel, who I learned was going to be running national events. I'd be happy if I could get close to them on my first time at the track. But every time I thought I had an open track and a chance to turn a quick lap, I would come across the #24 kart again and struggle to get past him. I could pass drivers who were *faster* than him, yet #24 was a puzzle I couldn't solve. Frustration set in. On one of these encounters, I caught him as we approached turn three. I had built up momentum through turns one and two and attacked him on the inside. But I misjudged the entry, ramped over the apex curb, and found myself in a four-wheel flight over the track.

Karts have no suspension to speak of, and the hard landing sucked the breath from my lungs. I did several spins in the grass before regaining control. The engine was still running, so I drove back to the pits with mud all over my kart, and we loaded everything for the trip home.

Even with my troubles with #24, it had been a great day. As we left the track, my dad asked, "Did you have fun?"

I just grinned. My dad stared at me and *kept* staring. When I asked why, he said, "Aaron, you have so much grass in your teeth!"

I looked in the mirror, saw the flecks of green, and smiled even more.

A great day? This was heaven.

The First Race

IT WAS 5:00 A.M. ON WHAT WAS GOING TO BE A COOL, humid April day. I didn't need to be out of bed for two more hours, but I couldn't sleep. It was finally race day. My dad was shocked to find me already awake when he got up. Hey, when you've looked forward to something for so long and it's finally here, sleep is the last thing on your mind.

When we left the house, the sunlight was breaking through the clouds and burning away the morning mist. Once again, we stopped for donuts. I told my dad I was too nervous to eat, and he reminded me, as parents do, that starving children around the world would do anything to have a nice breakfast. I took that to heart and worked my way through two glazed donuts.

It had been a long road, but all my anticipation was about to be put to rest. We pulled into the track and stopped at the pit gate. As my dad filled out the paperwork, I looked out at the track. The grass was neatly trimmed and hay bales now lined the turns. The ground was soft from last week's rain; walking around was like stepping on sponges, with water and mud seeping up from the ground. My dad called me over to sign some papers, and as I put the release form back on the table, the lady there asked me, "So, today's your first race?"

Enthusiastically, I replied, "Yes, and I can't wait!" "Well then, enjoy yourself," she said. "Have fun, and don't worry about how you do."

Enjoy myself? I wasn't here to enjoy myself. I was here to win, or at worst finish in the top five.

We pulled into the pits and emptied the van. Most of the other teams were pulling their karts out of nice trailers, but all of our equipment, kart included, was stuffed into dad's Ford Aerostar. By the time we got unloaded, just about ten minutes remained before practice.

I got into my suit, helmet, and rib protector, and lined up in a group of other karts. When the track announcer gave the call for my division, out we went. The last time we were at the track, the weather had been warm, but today the cooler temps limited the grip in the tires, just like in that cold 1992 Indy 500. Right away, my kart spun like a top. I didn't hit anyone or anything, but I felt foolish. I beat myself up through the rest of the session, even though I was fast enough to pass many of the karts I would later be racing.

After one more practice session, it was time for the drivers' meeting. The race director talked for a while, and then the flagman, a thin fellow who looked to be in his 70s, told everyone how he wanted the karts aligned when they came to the start. After the meeting, the race director met with all the rookie drivers to go over the race procedures. He explained the flags and how the program would work: There'd be two heat races and then a feature race. He told us that for our first three race weekends, all rookies would start in the back for safety reasons. Then he said, "And remember, it's your first race. Don't be concerned with how you do. Just have fun."

Everyone kept saying that: "Have fun!" Did they not know I was out for a top-five finish, maybe a win? It was driving me up a wall. Hadn't I always won in the video games I played?

Twenty minutes after the drivers' meeting, it was time for my first real competition, the heat race. We started our engines and waited. My mind began racing ferociously. I thought about the insurance papers saying that severe injury or death could occur. I thought about what my mom said as I left the house: "Now, Aaron, whatever you do, just don't get hurt. You hear me? Don't get hurt." In minutes, I'd be traveling over 40 miles per hour without a seatbelt or a roll cage in a kart that sat two inches off the ground. Not the safest activity for a 12-year-old. My mind raced around like a dog chasing its tail until we got the signal to roll.

As soon as I started picking up speed, every thought about danger vanished. We did one warm-up lap, and then it was time to get serious. I was starting 15th out of 17, and as we rolled off the final corner, I saw the green flag. It was one of the most nerve-racking moments in my life; there was a kart behind me, a kart beside me, and 14 karts in front of me. As we entered turn one, a couple of karts ahead of me tangled and spun. Oh no, I thought, I might get hurt after all. What's my mom going to think? But I made a great move, avoided the two pirouetting karts, and advanced to eighth place.

The late Allen Barklage—a local TV helicopter pilot who died years later in a chopper crash—was the SLKA announcer. By lap four out of 10, I had moved up to second and was challenging for the lead. I went for the lead going into turn one, and even in the kart I could hear Barklage's enthusiasm: "That's Aaron Likens challenging the leader, Justin Rodriguez. Side by side they go. Oh, they've touched, and Aaron's going to spin! Whoa, he saved it. How did he save that? I can't believe this is only Aaron's first race."

I didn't quite pull off the pass, but I had another chance on the final lap. Barklage commented, "Coming out of the final turn, Aaron to the inside, for the lead! Nope! Not going to get the win, but a valiant effort for just his first race."

As I pulled off the track and onto the scales for the mandatory weigh-in, everyone gave me the thumbs-up sign and clapped. The feeling was indescribable, and the look of disbelief on my dad's face was priceless. I'm sure he thought I'd do okay, but I don't think he was expecting me to battle for the race win. As we lifted the kart onto the scale, I asked him, "How'd I do?" My dad did not reply. He appeared to be in a state of shock.

In the next heat race, I finished fifth. In hindsight, that was still impressive, given my lack of experience. But, having finished second in the earlier heat, I was disappointed. My results in the heat races would normally have entitled me to start third in the feature, but as a rookie I would again be back in 15th.

It was getting late in the day. The sun was now in the western part of the sky, and clouds had drifted in. Ten minutes before the feature, I asked my dad, "How do you think I'll do?"

"You'll do just fine," he replied.

"Are you sure?"

"Absolutely," he said calmly.

It turned out I did do well. I finished fourth in the main

event, making for an excellent day overall. As we headed home, I asked my dad again, "So, Dad, how'd I do?"

"Well," he responded, "let's just say you've got it. Someday, you're going to win the Indianapolis 500."

Wow! I thought: Maybe I do have it.

Right then, I decided that racing would be my career. That would be Plan A for my life. There was no Plan B. Nothing would keep me from my dream.

The Perils of Early Success

THE PRESSURE TO WIN AFTER SUCH AN IMPROBABLE START was immense. That first heat race was a rush I had never experienced; finishing second from so far back, as a rookie, meant that winning would soon be commonplace, right? Well … as with so much in my life, there's a problem with being good right from the start.

It was the same problem in school: If I conquered something right away, I expected everything to come just as quickly. But that's not how life works, and that's certainly not how racing works because every other driver has the same goal.

Most of the races from that first year are cloudy to me now. I remember more about being *at* the track, rather than *on* the track. I befriended the driver of the #24 kart and his family, hoping that he might cut me a break when we were racing, but that didn't work.

And I remember countless ways in which I avoided having to change my own engine oil. I knew it was due to be changed after "X" number of laps, so when we were close, I resorted to counting my laps. Then I became a chameleon, disappearing and blending in elsewhere. I might be playing with other kids at the river's edge or having lunch with #24 and his family. But most of the time, I'd be standing in turn five, serving as a volunteer corner worker with a yellow flag.

It was my first time using a full-sized flag, and I still can't believe they let a 12-year-old do it. But there I was at oil-change time, working turn five. When my dad had the kart ready, he would come out and join me. On one occasion, he taught me a lesson I have never forgotten.

Working turn five could be precarious because if a kart spun off in turn four, it was possible that you could be hit. This was a busy area of the track; turn five was a long left-hander with a history of accidents. On this one day, a kart spun on the exit of turn five, so I walked right to the edge of the track, waving the flag and walking with my back to traffic. As the karts passed, I felt gravity disappear; I thought I'd been hit by a kart. Then I recognized the feeling of my father's hands on my ribcage, lifting me. He spun me around, got on one knee, and yelled over the engines, "Aaron, don't you *ever* turn your back to traffic!"

That's just common sense, but I learned that lesson because of the forceful tone my dad used. *Always* be aware; *never* turn your back to traffic.

Meanwhile, the frustration of not ending up in victory lane was wearing on me. You could count on me to finish in the top five, but cracking the top 3 was not happening.

At each event, there was a random pill draw for starting positions in heat one; for heat two, that lineup was reversed. In theory, your luck in a random draw should average out over the course of a season, but, as they say, theory never won a race. I had a great talent for drawing in the middle of the pack, so even heat-race wins were very hard to come by.

Now it was a sweltering day in mid-September, and the next-to-last race of the season. For once, I got a good draw.

I just missed winning the first heat race and made my way up in the second heat after starting near the back. That gave me a front-row starting spot for the feature. This was my chance. I wanted a win, and if that meant taking extra risks, so be it.

To this point, I had never spun out another kart, intentionally or otherwise. I was the epitome of a clean driver because I had a fear of being black-flagged for being too aggressive. At times, other drivers got away with spinning *me* out, but I was sure I'd be called out.

Starting outside the front row, I got a good start. The pole-position driver and I went side by side through turns one, two, three, four, and even tricky turns five and six. Turn seven was a flat-out right-hander, and taking the inside line was vital to have the proper angle into the next corner. I was almost fully past the other driver, but in my peripheral vision I could still see the sunlight reflecting off his front bumper, which meant that part of his kart was still beside me on my right. I used an aggressive racing tactic. I turned into the corner, giving him two options: back out of the throttle and concede the position, or have a collision that might force us both out. But he was as hungry as I was, and our karts touched, with his left-front wheel hitting my right rear.

I could feel the kart get light; I turned hard left, but my kart was in the air, so my steering inputs were futile. The world went into slow motion as I spun, and then sped up again as other karts started hitting mine. I felt like a pinball bouncing around inside its machine.

I could see concerned faces in the tech area in the pits, because this crash was the type of "big one" that you see in the final laps of a Daytona 500. Most of the field was collected, and I was bumped and banged all the way into the hay bales that protected the pit exit. As I stopped, I glanced behind me and saw one go through a brutal series of quick flips. Watching this, I regretted having been so aggressive.

The race was red-flagged, and a complete restart was ordered. My cutthroat style vanished, and I fell through the running order like a boat anchor. Later, I complained to my dad that maybe the alignment had been knocked out in the crash, but the truth was that I wasn't the same driver I'd been earlier in the day.

I got over it and returned to form, but I had learned another lesson: Early success creates an expectation that great results will come automatically, but that's not how life works. Early success does not guarantee further success.

Aaron, Meet Frankie

IT WAS THE LAST RACE OF THE YEAR, AND I WAS RUNNING out of safe havens to avoid changing oil. Working turn five was not an excuse on this occasion, because our pit stall was close enough that my dad could wave me over between races. I needed a plan that put me farther away.

Remember the flagger I mentioned earlier, the thin gentleman in his 70s? His name was Frankie Neidenbach. I still had a love of waving flags, so I volunteered to help Frankie when I wasn't racing. I expected a "no," but I was given a radio and told that I was Frankie's assistant.

Frankie's initial reaction was, well, gruff. Maybe he thought I was being groomed to replace him. But I was cheerful and never overstepped my bounds, and the curtness he showed earlier vanished by the lunch break. He said he'd been starting races since the end of World War II. He'd mostly worked at motorcycle events, but had also flagged boat races, Midgets, and Sprint Cars. I told him about my Duane Sweeney flag, which he thought was special. After I told him that story, he let me wave the white flag for the last race of our season.

—— It's all Good, until it's Not ——

THE 1995-96 OFF-SEASON WAS LONG AND BEING HOMESCHOOLED made it seem even longer yet. I'm not sure if it was the painful wait to get back behind the wheel or the prospect of furthering my role as assistant starter to a man with 50-plus years of racing experience, but the winter dragged on. Finally, the snow melted, and the '96 season brought a big change: At 13, I was now considered a "junior" driver. That meant a larger restrictor plate, which meant more horse-power, and wider rear tires, which meant a faster kart. And I kept my job as assistant starter, so all oil changes were too far away for me to help.

Frankie was glad to see me again, and I was glad to see him. Sadly, that's my best memory of him. I struggle to remember what people look and sound like, and in this case that saddens me. This man truly opened a door for me and is a big part of my story, yet he is remembered in shadows. But I've done some research, and I found a photo of Frankie from a race in 1954. I like to think of him as he appears in that photo, young and in his prime.

Over the first three races in 1996, I struggled on track but had a blast helping Frankie. He let me flag a heat race or two each week, which lessened the pain of running mid-pack in my new class. Running a more powerful engine against more experienced rivals was a kick in the teeth; I was always at least three positions away from trophy territory. My dad and I tried radical setup changes, but we always seemed to end up a tenth of a second off the leader's pace. A tenth is the blink of an eye, but in racing it can be the difference between a good day and a great one.

By mid-season the Meramec River overflowed its banks, but the club had a backup plan, moving our events to Gateway International Raceway, just across the Mississippi River in Madison, Illinois. Gateway—today known as World Wide Technology Raceway—was a much different facility before the current oval track opened in 1997. It had a drag strip and a 1.5-mile road course that was made available to our club. Obviously, this was much faster than our .35-mile layout at Widman County Park. Gateway was so fast that a kart could draft in the slipstream of the one just ahead; in fact, drafting became a key part of our racing there. And the corners were so wide that only one required a driver to lift the throttle. This was as close to flat-out racing as I had ever experienced. Right away, three and four-wide racing was commonplace.

With higher speeds come greater risks, and I was not allowed to help with flagging at Gateway. Frankie worked from a position between guardrails, and it was felt that any crash at that point on the straightaway might be a problem if two flagmen had to scramble for safety. I tried to argue that I was more agile than Frankie, but my dad shushed me. It was not open to debate.

Though disappointed about the flagging situation, I loved the flat-out racing. The sense of speed wasn't too high because the track was so wide, but the closeness of the racing got my adrenaline flowing. My first Gateway heat race was a great one; I came out of mid-pack and found myself fighting for second. Coming to the line I was in third, pressing the second-place kart, and when I looked to my left, I was being challenged by the driver in fourth. But I made a slick move: I jumped off the throttle so I could use the draft from *both* their karts, and it worked exactly as planned. I passed them both just before we got the checkered flag. Second place was a great result and would set me up for a nice grid spot in the feature if I had a good second heat.

I started toward the rear in heat number two. Right in front of me was my old nemesis, the #24 kart, which was also slow at this track. Passing him should've been easy on this wide track, but when I tried him on the inside, I almost had my kart's nose chopped off. I jumped off the throttle and watched the rest of the field inching away. To have any chance of a good finish, I needed to stay in their draft.

Heading into the only corner that required any bit of slowdown, I saw another kart, #64, get a bit out of shape. It slid to the left, right, left, right, until the driver finally lost control and spun. I was sure it was going to collect several other karts, but somehow, they all missed him. He had spun off-line, so, anxious not to lose ground to the pack, I stayed wide open, full throttle. "He's out of the way," I told myself. "I should be good."

Well, "should be good" can fade quickly when you're racing. Focused on his kart, I missed my turn-in point by a few feet, which put me off-line. This corner was off camber, meaning the track sloped *away*; think of it as the opposite of a banked turn. That made this corner extremely tricky; even more so because I was running off-line.

As I neared the scene, I swore the #64 kart started inching toward my line. Alarmed, I put a little bit more steering into my kart and started to skid. That's when the impact occurred.

At 60 or so miles per hour, my left-front side panel hit the nose of his kart. That sent my kart into a helicopter-type spin; I might have been ejected from the seat were it not for the fact that my kart's side panel was now lodged against my ribcage.

I don't recall the actual impact, but I remember regaining my senses and seeing the ambulance, which happened to be parked at this corner. I hit the throttle, thinking I could just drive away, but instead my kart sort of spun in place. I had no idea why it wouldn't move until I looked down and saw the sidepod bodywork wedged into the left rear wheel.

That's when I tried to take my first breath, and there was nothing there. Remember that panel jammed into my ribs? My wind had been forced out of my lungs, and the pain was intense. When I tried to yell, there was nothing. I never panicked, not even when I saw the EMTs climb out of the ambulance and head straight for me.

It took some force for them to bend the sidepod enough for me to get out of the kart. While this was happening, the field came past us, which triggered my racing brain: I wanted to get back in the seat of my kart and go! I had to be reminded that I had crashed, hard, and that I had to walk with them to the back of the ambulance to get checked out.

It was suggested that I get an X-ray to see if my spleen was okay, which I later did. The spleen was fine, but the crash had a lasting psychological effect. I began racing scared. There's nothing more dangerous for a driver than being afraid because you'll start second-guessing every move. The best drivers rely on instinct, and overthinking a situation is the opposite of instinct. Waste time overthinking, and you'll find yourself driving *behind* where you are on track. Also, drivers expect one another to make decisive moves, so any hesitation on your part can throw off what *they're* doing. Often, the result of racing scared is the very thing causing the fear: crashing.

For a couple of seasons, I had incident after frustrating incident. All the success and pride I took from my earliest races were now distant memories. Perhaps this racing thing wasn't going to be my thing after all.

The Story of Vegas 1996: An Intruder in the Garage and Breakfast with Bobby Unser

WHILE MY ASPIRATIONS TO ONE DAY RACE AT INDIANAPOLIS were still in my mind, my dad made it to the IndyCar series in another way. He'd done some video work for VisionAire, an upstart business-jet company, and was good friends with the owner, Jim Rice. VisionAire was in the process of raising millions of dollars to bring their single-engine business jet to market. My dad told Jim that he knew Jonathan Byrd, owner of the largest cafeteria in America, who also had an IndyCar team. My dad arranged a meeting between Jim and Jonathan and a sponsorship deal was put together. Vision-Aire would use the sponsorship to both find investors and market its jet, called the Vantage. The first race under this arrangement came in September of 1996 at the new Las Vegas Motor Speedway, and my dad and I were there.

We got to Vegas several days early so my dad could travel to Mojave, California, to tape an interview with Burt Rutan, the legendary airplane designer who'd built the first Vantage. We also attended the gala introduction of the new IndyCar chassis that was to debut in 1997. At that function, there were several Sega Indy 500 arcade games, and I went on a winning streak. One player walked away muttering,

"Damn kid!" I found out later that it was 1996 Indy Racing League champion Buzz Calkins.

The first day at the track was a trial for me. At 13, I didn't qualify for entry into the garage area, where my dad was working. However, rather than have me roaming the grounds, it was decided that I could be in the garage area as long as I stayed in a vehicle. I was relegated to sitting in our rental van. Las Vegas was in the middle of a triple-digit heat wave, and even with the air conditioner running full blast, it was intensely hot inside the van. Sweat dripped from my forehead. At one point, I gently honked the horn to get my dad's attention.

Jonathan Byrd looked my way, and my dad explained the situation. Jonathan motioned for me to exit the van, waved me into the garage. Was I nervous? You bet! But Jonathan calmed me down. He said, "I hear you have to stay in a vehicle if you're going to be in the garage area, so how about sitting in the race car?"

This team held the record for the fastest single qualifying lap and the fastest four-lap average at Indianapolis for 26 years. The driver, Arie Luyendyk, won the 1990 Indy 500 and was the driver who would've received the checkered flag that Duane Sweeney gave to me. Did I want to sit in their car? Mr. Byrd didn't have to ask me twice.

I was made to feel like I was part of the team. The crew members had me turn the steering wheel while they checked the alignment. I'm sure the grin on my face was huge. At one point a series official approached, and Jonathan motioned for me to hide. I sank into the cockpit and remained hidden.

It was much cooler in the race car, literally and figuratively, than in the van, but it came time to leave. When I'd climbed into the car, a crewman attached the steering wheel after I was in the seat; now that they were signaling me to climb out, I was unsure how to detach it. Jonathan said, "It's a quick-release wheel. Just grab the collar on the back of it and pull." I tugged, but it wouldn't budge. He said, "It's not *that* hard." Afraid that I was losing points with a team own-er who might one day need my driving talents, I squeezed the collar and pulled with all my strength. Whoever coined the term "quick release" was not kidding; the wheel, still in my hands, slid off the steering shaft and right into my face. I was dazed.

Jonathan was concerned. Not concerned that I might have just suffered a concussion, but instead concerned that his whole "sitting in a vehicle" loophole might be exposed. He leaned over me and he said, "Aaron, I don't care if your arm is broken or your leg is hanging off, you are *not* hurt. Got it? *You are not hurt!*" Thankfully, there were no inju-ries, minus my pride. I climbed from the car without being discovered, and without finding another way to hurt myself.

A day or too later, my inability to hang out in the garage area was not so bad, because the Byrd team's hospitality tent was now set up. There was shade, as well as a buffet. While I was eating breakfast, Bobby Unser, the three-time Indy 500 winner and legendary TV commentator, came in and sat down. I always tensed up around anyone with a hint of fame. How is one supposed to act? Are you supposed to acknowledge a legend like Bobby, or let the moment pass? I decided to avoid eye contact, but my hopes of staying invis-ible were dashed when he moved from his table to mine. He sat beside me and asked, "Son, do you like racing?"

I tried to find words. It should've been easy with a question like that, but this was *Bobby Unser* asking. Quietly, I said, "Yes, I do." With a quick-fire response, he said, "Do you want to race when you grow up?" This perked me up because I proudly responded, "I race *now*," and mentioned my karting. He added, "How did you do in your last race?"

The week before Las Vegas, my performance had improved. I was battling for the lead in the feature, my heart was soaring at the thought of a new trophy for the collection, when my kart went into a wild spin. My right-rear wheel had fallen off, and my chance of victory was gone.

I mentioned to Bobby that the wheel had come off because my dad forgot to tighten it. He stopped me and said, "Son, if you want to make it in racing or in life, you've got to learn this one lesson: Never, and I mean never, criticize those on your crew. At the end of the day, they're the ones who tighten all the bolts, and if you don't support them, they won't support you. This goes for outside racing, too. It's a lesson you must learn."

Bobby had a unique way of speaking, and if you were familiar with it, you may have "heard" him delivering that short speech to me.

I was unsure how to react, so I just stared forward, processing his words. I had no idea that what I'd just done was a taboo in the racing world. How could I ever recover from this?

But Bobby broke the silence. He said, "What could you have done to prevent it? Aren't you part of the crew as well?" This gave me a chance to explain that while the kart was being prepared for the feature, I'd been across the track working as the assistant flagman. Then I mentioned the flag given to me by Duane Sweeney, and Bobby lit up. I asked if he would sign it, because I had a goal of getting it autographed by Indy 500 winners, and he did that for me.

With the life lessons out of the way, we talked about racing for 30 minutes. With every second, my shyness disappeared more. He was no longer a legend on an unreachable pedestal, but a human being with a passion for racing, a passion that I understood very well.

I often think back to my breakfast with Bobby. Just as Duane Sweeney gave me a flag that helped me along my path, Bobby gave me advice that I could use in almost any situation. The concept of "What could *you* have done" is vital everywhere. Instead of blaming others for whatever went wrong, find the positive steps that you can take to make things better.

Bobby Unser passed away in May of 2021. Even as an adult, I cried when I heard the news. I don't pick up on many emotions from other people, but passion is an unmistakable thing. Those 30 minutes of sharing breakfast and passion with Bobby are something I'll cherish for the rest of my life.

Solo for the First Time

SPRING RAINS AND FLOODING IN 1997 AGAIN MADE RACING at Widman impossible. Watching the news to learn when the rivers would crest became a daily event, one I began to hate; they kept pushing their predictions back, meaning another week or month that I wouldn't be racing. I remembered hearing about the lost season in 1993 and wondered if I'd ever race again.

But again, the club found an alternative. This time it was a track in West Quincy, Missouri, a tiny town just across the Mississippi River from Quincy, Illinois.

I still remember our first drive north to race there. It took more than two hours and made me imagine that this was like *professional* racing because there was travel involved. Of course, NASCAR and IndyCar drivers like Mark Martin or Al Unser Jr. weren't traveling in Ford Aerostar vans with all their equipment—and in our case, the race vehicle, too—stuffed in the back. But as a race-hungry 14-year-old, I felt as if I was discovering a new world.

The kart track in West Quincy is one of the oldest in America, and just the third track I'd driven on, which was exciting. It was even more exciting learning the final corner was called "Monza," named for the famous old high-banked track in Italy.

My dad had hired a co-worker, who also owned a quilting shop, to make me a set of flags almost identical to Duane Sweeney's. They were finished just a couple weeks before our first race at West Quincy, where I looked forward to once again helping Frankie when I wasn't racing. Instead, after our Saturday practice day came and went, I was given some surprising news: The kart club would not pay Frankie to drive up there and flag the races, and they were counting on me to take his place. The nerves set in quickly. I was 14. Sure, I'd had more than a full season helping Frankie, but he always handled the split-second decisions; I'd only been there to assist him. Now, at a track I'd never even seen, I'd be in charge.

On Sunday morning, the race director talked to me. We'd never had a one-on-one discussion, and I suppose he wanted to make sure I knew what I was doing. Whatever he was looking for out of that conversation, I passed the test. I took my new flags—along with a special holder my dad had made—and walked to the start/finish line. I was more nervous than when I first drove my kart. My pulse throbbed in my neck, wrists, and feet. Even though at this track I was protected by a sturdy flagstand, I felt more exposed than at any race I'd been involved in. When I was driving, I could control my kart, which gave me a strong sense of steering my own destiny. And if I screwed up behind the wheel, it was more than likely just me getting hurt; if I messed up on the flagstand—waved the wrong flag, or made some other mistake—the consequences could be serious, even tragic. I was almost overwhelmed.

Yet when the karts rolled from the grid, and I was alone in my "office," my hyper-focus set in. Everything felt natural. I had the yellow flag rolled up in my left hand, and the green flag behind my right leg, the same stance I've always used ever since.

It's impossible to fully describe how quickly I went from fearing this moment to commanding the position of chief starter. I could use a cliché—"a light switch turned on," or some such thing—but that wouldn't cover it.

The dozen or so karts made it through turns six and seven, and the front row got to the final Monza corner. The front row looked good, going nice and slow, and in proper alignment. I got into a ready position with my legs firmly planted and my head hunched forward, ready to unleash the green. Slowly, *slowly*, the karts crept towards me. I liked this. I liked it a lot.

I had only waved the green in a couple of heat races when working with Frankie, but I knew a good start when I saw one. "Just a bit closer," I thought to myself. This was it! I was ready to go ... and then I heard on the radio, "Yellow, yellow! No start, no start!"

I quickly displayed the yellow flag. Had I done something wrong? That self-doubt came back in a flood. Then, over the radio, came the race director's voice: "Sorry, I thought there were still a couple karts left on the grid, but they're just getting ready for the next race."

It was a reminder that if I wanted this job, I'd have to be ready for anything.

After one more pace lap, and with the pack of karts again nicely aligned, I waved the green flag. The sound of accelerating engines mixed with the flapping of the flag in my hand was the most incredible sensation I had ever felt. With each start that day, I felt more confident. In one of the feature races, a kart flipped in the Monza corner and my instincts took over. Without direction from the race director, I waved the red flag and stopped the race. I smiled inside, satisfied with my reaction under pressure.

My quick actions drew kudos from the race director and

the scorekeepers, and as the day ended, I wondered what the future held. I don't recall how I finished in the races I drove that day, but I'd been given a chance to shine in another capacity, and I did. I also made $25 for flagging. Little did anyone know that I would have gladly paid more than that for the opportunity.

Meeting Duane

MAY 1997. THANKS TO MY DAD'S CONNECTION WITH THE Byrd team, we went to the Indianapolis Motor Speedway for qualifying. I brought the flag Duane Sweeney had given me, hoping to get more 500 champions to autograph it. Right away, I saw three-time winner Johnny Rutherford, and he signed it. That was my first big thrill of the day, but my dad had another one planned. We walked toward the south end of the track and went through a gate. I began to panic, thinking we were in a restricted area where I wasn't supposed to be. My dad assured me it was fine. We went around a corner, and there, sitting in a golf cart, was Duane Sweeney. I froze.

What was I going to say? I'd never sent him a thank-you letter. I wanted to but had no idea how to write one. Should I now say, "Hi, I'm Aaron, and you gave me a priceless relic that I never thanked you for," or, "Hi, I'm the kid you gave a flag to," or something else? Although I had dreamed of this moment, my nerves made me want to be somewhere else.

Duane was talking with Bryan Howard, who took over the chief starter's role in 1998, so he hadn't yet noticed me and my dad standing there. I was holding my breath.

A few more seconds passed. My eyes were darting everywhere but in Duane's direction. As in my breakfast with Bobby Unser, I had no idea how to deal with anyone I deemed famous.

"Mr. Sweeney," said my dad, breaking the ice. "Mr. Sweeney, thanks to JoAnn Petrie you gave my son one of your checkered flags in 1990, and we thank you very much for that. But you signed it for 'Erin' rather than 'Aaron,' and we were hoping you could re-sign it."

Duane looked at me, and as I reached out to hand him the flag, there were so many words I wanted to say. He was a true childhood hero who'd given me one of the rarest pieces of racing memorabilia, and something that meant the world to me, yet I stayed silent.

Inside my head, my brain was displaying the most lavish fireworks show in the world, and I tried to think of things I wanted to tell him: "Mr. Sweeney, thanks so much!" … "Mr. Sweeney, or Duane, can I call you Duane? I've used your flag in real races!" … "Duane, my future self is already regretting this moment, because your kind deed set a path for me, yet someday I'm going to look back and cry at my inability to talk to you."

It's true, even as he re-signed the flag, I was already thinking about how I'd look back on this moment. I hadn't yet been diagnosed on the autism spectrum, but I knew something about me was different, because despite mustering every bit of courage I had, all I could do was whisper, at a barely audible level, "Thank you."

In life, we all have chance meetings, and if we're one of the rare and lucky few, we'll meet the people who changed our lives. Maybe we'll be able to genuinely convey our gratitude, or maybe, like me, the right words will dry up like raindrops in a desert. I look back on meeting Mr. Sweeney with a level of regret I haven't experienced with any other event. Of course, how could I know then that the destiny I envisioned that day would come true? I was only an awkward 14-year-old who struggled with basic conversation. Should I still carry the regret as I do? Or do my actions and deeds as an adult offset that awkward youngster's inability to speak up or write a letter? Even now, I wonder about this.

A Lesson Given in the Agony of Defeats

BACK HOME, THE FLOODING CONTINUED INTO THE SUMMER of '97, and the St. Louis Karting Association might well have been renamed the Quincy-Area Kart Club, with as much time as we spent there. On the bright side, I was proving that I could handle my role as sole starter. I was also growing more comfortable in the job. For example, I thought the starter should always know the lap count in case a radio failed, or the scorers got distracted, so my dad bought a tally counter that I attached to my belt loop. I clicked it each time the field passed, and at a glance I knew what lap we were on.

Unfortunately, my on-track performance was still in a valley. I always seemed to be in the wrong place at the wrong time. One week, I jumped to the outside of another kart heading into turn three, and I suspected that the driver beside me had no idea I was there. In racing, this is a version of no-man's land, because if he doesn't know you're there and moves over into your lane, you both might crash. Lifting off the throttle would have been the wise play for me, but I was frustrated so I held my ground. Sure enough, the other kart moved toward mine, the contact lifted the nose of my kart, and I went flying off into the weeds. I was furious.

I jumped out of the kart to push it back on track, but at 14, I was exceptionally scrawny and had no brute strength.

The race director hurried over to assist. Once the kart was back on track, I should have jumped back into the seat, but I kept pushing. He screamed at me, "Get in the f***ing kart!"

Whoa! I was frozen, trying to assess what had just happened. My parents had taught me that this type of language is, unequivocally, never allowed. *Never.*

The race director was pointing at me to *GO!* as my kart sat stationary on the racing line. Eventually, the rest of the pack made its way past us. Finally, I took off, but I was a lap down.

I kept the story of the race director's language to myself as long as I could. Several days later, riding in the car with my dad, I broke down and laid it all out. My dad listened, and then said, "Aaron, do you think there are exceptions to rules?"

I exclaimed, "Absolutely not!"

He responded, "Do you think he was trying to hurt you, or your feelings?"

I didn't have much of an answer. Not skipping a beat, he said, "Did it get your attention?"

I was angry. "Of course it did!"

"Getting your attention so you would do what he wanted was his intent," my dad said. "He didn't want to hurt you. If he did, do you think he'd have run over to help you back on track? Would he have risked hurting himself while pushing you back on track if he wanted to hurt you?"

I shook my head. *Maybe* there were times when it was okay to break a rule.

My dad explained that there were times when people would use inappropriate words in heated moments, or in emergencies. And, since racing was full of heated moments and passion, I might hear those words a lot. He was not wrong about that.

The next time we went to West Quincy, I spun out early

in my first practice session on the day before the race. Yes, it was in turn three. Was I spooked because of the previous week's episode with the race director? The next lap, I spun there again, and also spun in turn four. Hoping to correct the handling, my dad made wholesale changes to the kart, but it was to no avail. It must have looked like I was practicing 360-degree spins.

Back in the pits, having run out of ideas to change on the kart itself, we took a good look at the tires. The wear indicators were gone, meaning the tire had no remaining life, and that equates to zero grip. Imagine your car in heavy rain, on tires without tread; that's pretty much the feeling I had. Karting at this level isn't like the upper tiers of racing, where teams constantly bolt on a new set of tires; the ones we ran were meant to last up to half a season, and we had used up that half-season. The trouble was, my dad had left the new tires in the garage.

We loaded the kart into the van and checked into the Holiday Inn across the river in Quincy, Illinois. Then my dad drove home to St. Louis, grabbed a set of new tires, and made it back to the hotel after a four-hour round trip. That is dedication.

The next day I was fast, or at least faster than I had been. In practice, I passed karts that had previously been able to pull away from me. I could feel my confidence coming back.

The pill draw didn't go my way—again—so the heat races were going to be tough. Since my big crash I'd been timid about passing, but on this day, I was going for it in places where I didn't know I could overtake. Three times, I drafted other karts down the main straightaway, darted outside them just as the drivers feathered the throttle for turn one, and took the long way around. I'd never seen anyone even *attempt* an outside pass there, but I made it work each time.

Heading into the 14-lap feature, I knew I was competing for a trophy for the first time in ages. Finishing in the top five was the target, and I was starting fifth; all I had to do was not lose a position. Sounds simple enough, right? But off the start, the kart in front of me didn't get up to speed right away, and I lost a position. The kart now just ahead of me was one I'd passed in the heat race with my new outside move in turn one, so I went for the same move. Once again, I swept around him and moved back into fifth place.

I talked to myself a lot in that race. I wanted a trophy so much it hurt; it had been over a year since I'd had a podium finish. "Ten to go, fourth is just ahead," I said. "Draft along and pull away from sixth. This will be easy!" But it got even better than that. I noticed that the fourth-place driver was also lifting into turn one. I don't think I had ever passed this guy in a main event, and I almost felt as if it wasn't my place to do so. But once again I jumped to the outside and smiled as I completed the pass before turn two.

"Okay, Aaron," said the voice in my head. "Third is about five seconds ahead. Where are the leaders?" They had driven away and were somewhere having a duel of their own.

As the substitute starter displayed crossed flags, the halfway sign, the third-place kart was creeping away from me. Where was fifth? I normally wouldn't look over my shoulder, because when you get too concerned about what's behind you, you can lose focus on where you're going. But curiosity got the best of me, and in the compound right-hand corners in the middle of the lap, I quickly turned my head; he was two corners back, no longer a worry.

Just then, the third-place driver put up his hand to warn others that he had a problem. Something mechanical had failed on his kart, and he pulled off. What a gift! Now I was third, well clear of fourth, and that shiny third-place trophy would be mine.

With four laps to go, I noticed my breathing becoming labored. Getting nervous over a third-place finish was absurd, but my drought of results and confidence had gone on for so long. Third was going to feel like a win. Then I saw the corner worker waving a yellow flag in turn two and noticed that two cars had spun off-track. Wait … those were the leaders!

I'd been hoping for fifth place, and now I was up front. I was leading on a day in which I'd made bold, decisive passes. Sure, first and second took each other out, but I had worked hard to be in a position to capitalize on their mistakes. Better yet, I had made no mistakes of my own.

Three laps to go, and then two, and then the white flag. I went through turn one and smiled at the passes I'd made there. In turn two, I avoided the menacing curb to the outside. I approached turn three, the scene of my drama with the race director. I reminded myself to be smooth, to hit my lines and bring it home …

Wait! What was that? Something that looked metallic flew over my right shoulder. Karts sometimes kick up rocks, but this didn't look like any rock.

When I hit the throttle to exit the corner, there was … nothing. Silence. I pumped the pedal, hoping, but there was no life in this kart. I looked down and saw that parts were missing from the front of the engine. That explained the metallic flash I'd seen.

I pulled to the side of the track, in shock. Other karts, their engines revving perfectly, went past, but I did not see them. I couldn't look anywhere but straight ahead, staring at the world but looking at nothing. Breathing felt almost impossible.

After that moment of shock, the emotion hit all at once. As the winner drove by, my eyes followed his kart with intense envy and filled with tears. Then, as the second-, third-, and fourth-place finishers rolled past me, I realized that I had to make it back to start/finish. I still had a job to do. The substitute flagger worked for the track and had to get back to his other duties. I left my kart and walked slowly across the track. My shoulders sagged as if gravity was pulling me down, but I kept walking.

I collected my green and yellow flags and my radio and was ready to get on with my flagging duties, albeit with depleted enthusiasm. Then a voice came over the radio; it was Terry Traeder, the track owner, who had been announcing the race.

He said, "Aaron, that sucked. I get it. When I raced, I had wins slip away like that, and it hurts. But there's no way to sugarcoat this: Aaron, you still have a job to do. You've got those flags in your hand. There will be setbacks like this in life. Everyone will have them, but it's how you bounce back that separates the back of the field from the champions. You already standing back at the start/finish line shows me you're a champion. So, finish out strong!"

I haven't received many pep talks like that, but Terry's words have stayed with me. A victory that day would have been sweet, but had I won, I'd have missed learning a critical lesson about the will to fight on, the obligation to finish the task at hand, and the fundamental need to bounce back and do the best damn job possible, even when gravity pulls you down.

For the final races that day, I stood with a firmer stance, and my flag-waving had an extra bit of kick to it. That victory could have been mine, but it wasn't, and I was okay with that. I was 14, and I'd have more chances.

Terry's words echoed in my mind, and I realized how lucky I was just to have a chance to fight for a win. And, more importantly, how lucky I was to be working at a track, finding my own niche in racing. The tears had faded, and by day's end I even had a bit of a smile.

A Season-Ending Crash

IT WAS THE AUTUMN OF 1997, AND THERE WERE THREE races left in the season, all at Widman County Park. My parents and I had dropped my homeschooling—temporarily, as you'll see—and I was enrolled in a parochial school midway through seventh grade. Now, in eighth grade, I found that sitting in classrooms could still be painful. It didn't help that the school pastor loathed that I was at a race track on Sundays instead of hearing his sermons. On Monday mornings, in front of my classmates, he'd say, "Aaron, where were you yesterday?" If I said that I was racing, he'd reply, "Thou shalt be at my service on Sundays. And thou shalt be hurt if you are at a track. Do you think God will protect you if you're not at my service?" I didn't let his words bother me. My dad was a pastor, and we prayed before the races, so I knew I was good in that department.

The next-to-last race came on a chilly day. And speaking of chills, my confidence level had cooled off now that we were back at our home track. I found myself again being timid at the wheel. Forget the outside passes I'd made at West Quincy; most of the passing I saw now consisted of other karts passing me.

I had a good pill draw and started the first heat from pole position but got off to a bad start and dropped through the field. In heat two I started last, but a big crash at the start knocked out several karts, giving me a decent finish. My heat results gave me a mid-pack start in the feature.

At the start of any race, anywhere, the middle of the pack is a tricky place to be. It's a bit of a crunch zone, prone to chain reactions, because the deeper you are in the running order, the more limited your vision is. Think of it this way: The leader is looking at a clear track, while you're busy dealing with all the action that's immediately around you. If there's a tangle up front, you might see it from your mid-pack position, but those behind you might not, and now they're piling into the back of you. It's a tough place to be until the field strings out a bit.

Coming off the final corner for the start, I was worried, almost scared. Something didn't feel right, and I almost wanted to pull out of the event. But I didn't, and the green flag flew. Then, just as I described, things started happening. The front-row karts touched wheels and bobbled, and immediately there was that chain reaction of some karts slowing down and others not recognizing the situation. All of us in the mid-pack slowed up, and here came the back of the field, with a run on us entering turn one, a moderately fast 90-degree right-hand corner.

I looked left, and there was a kart. I glanced right, and there was a kart. I knew I was in the middle of a three-wide formation, and then I caught a glimpse of blurred color beyond the kart to my right and realized that we were actually *four* wide. The track was wide enough for three, but four wouldn't work. I lifted off the gas, hoping to get out of trouble, but the others did the same; we had all done the smart, cautious thing, yet we were *still* four wide. The two karts on my right touched, pushing one of them into me, which ricocheted me into the kart to my left. The two of us hooked wheels and stopped. I hunkered down in the seat, expecting to be slammed from behind, but all the other karts missed us. I glanced down and saw that our front wheels were tangled, so I lifted myself out of the seat to help free my kart.

And that's when it happened. *BAM!*

Unbeknownst to me, there was an additional kart on the track. It was that driver's first race weekend, and he had been afraid to run in the heats but was allowed to tag along behind the field in the feature. It was a way for that driver to get some track time and be better prepared for the next event. So that kart was a fair distance behind us, which meant that after the main pack cleared the site of our two-kart incident, things went quiet for a moment, and I felt safe trying to get our karts untangled. Then this straggler kart arrived on the scene at full throttle; the driver may have also been lulled by target fixation and stayed on the throttle until that kart slammed into mine at full speed.

I'd never felt such an impact. The sound was sickening, and I found myself partially out of the seat, looking skyward, as my kart rolled down the track.

I settled back in the seat, grabbed the steering wheel, and pulled behind the hay bales between turns one and two. There I sat, and sat, and sat. The race continued as I attempted to regain my breath. I'd never had pain in my chest and my back that was anything like what I felt then. I was partially hidden behind the hay bales, and, besides, I'd obviously steered the kart there on my own, so no one would have guessed that I was hurt. Eventually, my dad, breaking protocol, ran to the scene. When he spoke to me, I tried to respond, but it hurt too much. The track medic, now sensing that something was amiss, hurried over and asked some questions. He must have thought I was okay because he had me drive my kart—which was undamaged except for the badly bent rear bumper—back to the pit area. My dad quickly loaded up the van, and we headed to a hospital.

The emergency-room staff took x-rays and other scans and found that I had a couple of cracked ribs, a slight fracture in one vertebra, and more than likely some damaged cartilage around my sternum. All internal organs were okay. I was told that I would hurt like hell for a while, maybe months, but there was nothing to be done except to let things heal.

The doctor didn't lie. It did hurt like hell.

A couple of weeks passed, and the missed school days added up. I couldn't sit upright in a chair for too long without ending up in tears from the pain.

About a month after the crash, I returned to class on a

Monday. A few kids asked what had happened to me, but the pastor was almost gloating.

"Aaron," he said, "do you remember what I told you?" I could see the game being played, and I was in *Zugzwang*, a chess term for being in a spot where the only available moves are all bad ones. If I said no, he'd tell me I was fibbing; if I said yes, he would ask why I hadn't heeded his warning.

He continued, "Aaron, your guardian angels weren't with you that day because you weren't at my service." Twisting doctrine to suit his own whims did not seem very Christian to me. He continued, "What do you suppose will happen the next time you're not at my church?"

I'd heard enough, and my ribs were hurting too much to handle my now-elevated breathing and heart rate. I clutched my ribs, and the teacher in the room sent me to the school nurse. I guess the pastor wanted to gloat some more, so he followed me into the small office, said a few things I didn't listen to, and then "accidentally" locked the door on his way out. The teacher seemed to feel that this was too much, that a line had been crossed, so I was sent home.

Shortly after that, my family went back to homeschooling, which to me was a giant step forward. All the drama with that pastor was a trying challenge.

As for my racing, I told myself I'd never be timid again. I would've been clear of those three karts beside me if I'd only stayed on the throttle. I suffered through a winter of pain, and I had a newfound determination to be at the front of the pack, unafraid.

A New Starter at Indy and Redemption on the Track

MUCH OF 1998 IS A BLUR TO ME. MY DAD AND I WERE AGAIN at Indy for qualifying. I saw that Bryan Howard was the new chief starter and that his style was very similar to Duane Sweeney's, which brought a smile to my face.

The 500 that year was on a cloudy, dreary day, but there was one bright pre-race moment when a dog ran two laps around the track and then detoured down the congested pit road. Track workers, safety personnel, and pit crew members tried to corral the dog, but this was his big day. He scurried through Purdue University's All-American Marching Band, then hurdled a guardrail and disappeared into the infield. That dog may have received the loudest cheers of the day.

As a racer, I was consistently in the fourth-through-seventh finishing range. I had drive and aggression, but there was always just a tenth of a second lacking to make it to the top three. I was getting agitated. Another driver innocently asked if maybe splitting my time between driving and flagging was hindering my speed. I looked at him, almost disgusted, and all I could say was, "No." How dare he make such an assumption? So, I didn't get a break all day from the summer heat and oppressive humidity of St. Louis in a sport that takes all of one's soul to be good at … wait, maybe he did have a point. But I wouldn't give it up.

In the buildup to the year's final race, the club announced that this would be the last time trophies would be handed out in all classes. The following year they would only be available for the juniors and the lower classes. This was my final race as a junior before I'd have to graduate to the adult classes, and suddenly it was also my last chance at a first-place trophy.

Saturday practice went well. My dad made a few setup

changes, and my lap times were the best they'd ever been. Race day came and the weather looked awful, with fog and a fine mist. I walked to turn one to watch the practice before my own session, and when I looked back, I could not see the final corner. This was a safety concern. But if we delayed things and started later than usual, the expected late-afternoon storms could wipe out the features, and there would be no makeup date if we had a washout. I might not have a chance at a trophy after all.

I started sixth in the feature. On speed alone, I knew I had a top-three kart. I strongly thought about jumping the start; after all, what would they do? The club did not issue post-race penalties, and the fill-in flagman likely wouldn't have the confidence to wave off the start. But imagine that, the regular chief starter willfully breaking the rules? I couldn't do it.

I did get an excellent start, though, and was fifth into turn one. By turn three, I was up to third. Just ahead was the driver who caused my worst crash; beyond him, the leader was a guy I'd competed with since my first race. I knew his moves, and I had a chance if I could get to him. It was a short race, though, just 12 laps, and the second-place driver was no easy overtake. I judged that it would be harder to overtake him than the leader. I was faster than both, but in racing the real art is not raw speed but passing.

We completed laps three, four, five, and then came the halfway sign, lap six. Each time I made a move on second, my rival countered. I could hear the fourth-place kart behind me. The leader was so far ahead that even if I took second, there probably wouldn't be enough laps left to battle for the win. But even a second-place trophy sounded great, so I hung tough.

It's uncanny how easy it is sometimes to find speed you didn't know you had, but it's also easy to lose speed. If you're closing on another kart, you might find a magical tenth of a second. But if that gap ahead of you starts to grow, the fight can be sucked right out of you, and you'll slow down without realizing it. I could not let this happen.

We were down to four laps remaining. I had to make this pass, and I had a plan. I would start the pass in turn three and keep crossing over; I'd have the inside for one corner, he'd have it the next, and so on, until we got to turn eight, the hairpin left, where I'd pass him for good.

Getting a perfect run out of turn two would make or break this maneuver, and I got one. I poked the nose of my kart far enough to his left that he saw me. The fight was on. As predicted, he had the line into four, then I had the run out of five. But one thing I hadn't counted on was a kart off in the grass to the right. Wait! That was the #27 kart, the leader! Suddenly, this fight for second was instead for the win, and I had the momentum to make a move.

The corner before the hairpin, I committed to go for it. Remember, go-karts have no mirrors, so I had to pull far enough alongside him that he saw me, or he'd cut me off, and if that happened my kart might ramp over his wheel and flip. The thought of what that might feel like flashed into my mind, but I brushed it aside. This was my only chance.

I held my breath as I cut under him. He turned in, and we bumped wheel to wheel, but we both maintained control. We fought hard through turns nine and ten, and I came out the leader.

Three laps to go. I had been this close before, only to have an engine issue. The race isn't over until the checkered flag waves and the finish line is crossed.

Into turn one, I heard him at my right-rear corner. He was coming back at me. Then he tried a desperation move and came up short. That hurt his momentum and allowed me to build a gap. At turn six, I couldn't hear him anymore. I hoped the fight had been sucked out of him.

A lap-and-a-half later, the white flag was displayed. It felt as if my entire life had played out just for this moment. Pressure? I don't think I took a breath for most of that last lap, and I was praying that I wouldn't see chunks of my engine fly off.

The cliché is true: Leading a race, close to the finish, you'll hear every rattle and feel every pebble you run over. I was two corners away. If everything held together, I had the win.

Around the final corner, I breathed once more. Through misty eyes, I saw Frankie's checkered flag twirling in the air. As I crossed the line, I stuck one hand into the air, and I screamed as loudly as possible. Through all the battles, the year or so of misery—injuries, the scorn from my school pastor—I had toughed it out. Now, finally, I had won.

After a brief embrace and some words with my dad, duty called. There were feature races for other classes yet to be run, and I was the chief starter. That was an odd way to celebrate a win, but there was work to do. I walked across the track to the flagstand.

And right there, beside my very own flags, the scorekeepers had set my very own first-place trophy.

I went to bed that night in a state of pure pride. It probably felt better to win after so many struggles than it would have if I'd won from the outset. I had dreamed big, and the dream came true. That night, I dreamed of something just a little bit bigger: crossing the yard of bricks at Indianapolis first after 500 miles.

A True Official?

NEWS CAME THROUGH THE GRAPEVINE THAT THE KARTING association was pushing Frankie into retirement. I had proven my worth, and no longer was the club afraid of a teenager—I was now 15—in control of the flags. I was elated, but sad at the same time. There would be no good-bye, and no public thank-you to Frankie. I tried to imagine being forced out that way, but I couldn't.

I was happy that he'd been there to wave the checkered flag over my first win.

It was going to be a bit odd working alone, but this was something I'd wanted. But I learned quickly that having the title of chief starter was no guarantee that all the adults would respect me. On opening day, there was a flip in one of the features. I threw the red flag, stopping the race. Before all the karts had even stopped, the driver who had flipped was walking towards me from turn one. He was uninjured, but his kart was probably destined for the scrapyard. I asked the man if he was okay, and he said, "I am, but that dirty driver has got to pay! He took me out, and no official will do anything about it."

I missed the social cue that should have told me this driver simply needed to vent.

Reflexively, to show him that someone was listening, I said, "*I'm* an official."

In response, he angrily commented, "Sorry kid, you're no f***ing official."

Once again, I was shocked by language, much like my earlier race-director episode. But I looked at this man's wrecked kart and thought about the fact that he appeared to be racing on a shoestring budget. I realized that his season may have ended after just a handful of laps. Yes, he violated the rules by directing language like that at an official—and I *was* an official—but I remembered my dad's lesson: It's okay sometimes to make exceptions to rules. There was no sense rubbing salt in this man's wound because he'd used rough language in a heated moment.

It's interesting how small events like this can condition us for the future. I learned not to pursue a conversation with an angry racer, because it might end badly. I also learned that my age was a disadvantage. People may have liked my flagging style, but I was years away from being respected as an authority figure.

—— 1999: The Start of the Second Act ——

IT'S ALMOST IMPOSSIBLE TO KNOW, IN REAL TIME, WHICH moments in life will be the ones that shape you. The same goes for recognizing, as you're passing through the mile markers we call years, exactly when you've exited one stage of your life and entered another. Looking back now, 1999 was a very significant crossing into the next stage of my life.

I was now chief starter of the St. Louis Karting Association, but that didn't mean I'd be working anytime soon. Again, the Meramec River had spilled over its banks. The season opener got pushed back repeatedly until it was decided that we'd start things off at West Quincy.

Riding up there for the opener on May 1, I was both elated and angry. Our season was about to begin, but I had really wanted to go to Charlotte for the VisionAire 500 Indy Racing League event. I had watched from VIP suites with my dad the previous two years, and we had grandstand tickets for the 1999 race. My dad and I planned to go. But he stressed to me the fact that I had obligations with the karting club, and more so now than ever because of my role as chief starter.

"You made a commitment," he said, "and you can't back out of it."

So, my racing season, and Act Two of my life, started on May 1 in West Quincy.

A Dark Day

AS WE UNLOADED THE KART FOR THE 1999 OPENER, MY expectations were high. My most recent result had been a win, so if you win once, surely you can win again and again, right? The top spot on the podium was no longer just a dream. I had been there. Of course, I would now be racing in an all-adult class, against drivers with many more years of experience.

I felt as if I had good speed in the first couple of practice sessions, but traffic was dense, and it was difficult to get a clean lap. A driver named Jeremy was frustrating me. Twice I passed him going into the banked Monza corner, and twice he passed me back on the exit. I couldn't understand why he didn't back off after I passed him, so we could both get clean laps.

Here's the absurd thing; *I* could've backed off, too, and looked for room enough to have a lap to myself. But once I got frustrated, I was determined to pass him and make it stick.

A couple of laps into the third practice session, Jeremy and I collided. My kart jumped into the air, and the world slowed down. It was moving frame by frame, slower than any replay you'll see in a sports broadcast. At one point, I looked down and saw Jeremy's arm being bent the wrong way between my seat and the side of my kart.

Out of control, the two of us entered the Monza corner. I went sliding over the top of the banking and into the tire barriers. I hopped out of the kart, unsure of how all of this had happened. The session had been stopped for our crash. My dad and Jeremy's dad—who was also an EMT—were sprinting to the scene. As they ran up, Jeremy's dad looked at my dad and screamed, "He came down on him! Why? He came down!"

I looked over at my dad, who had a profoundly concerned look on his face. Had I done something improper? Had I let him down by causing this crash?

I walked over to check on Jeremy, who was clearly in immense pain, favoring one arm. As his dad walked him away, I apologized; I wasn't sure I'd done anything wrong, but I didn't want him to be mad at me. Jeremy mumbled something I couldn't understand, and his dad took him to the hospital. He was back at the track later in the day, with a cast on his broken arm.

I skipped the next practice session, still shaken that I might have made a mistake that hurt someone, and I felt awful. I kept thinking of his dad yelling, "He came down!" Who was the "he" in that statement?

Thankfully, after Jeremy and his dad got back to the track, Jeremy's dad explained things. He was upset at watching Jeremy's kart come down into mine. I had held my line, and Jeremy, thinking he had more room, started a cross-over maneuver that resulted in our collision. The reality was, we were probably both at fault. Sometimes when helmets go on, brains turn off. We chose to battle it out in a *practice* session, with nothing at stake, and the result was Jeremy's broken arm and my realization that my actions could have hurt a competitor.

Our kart got loaded into the van after one more session. I needed a break from the track, and both my dad and I wanted to watch the Charlotte race on television. But after we checked into the hotel, we discovered that their cable package didn't include the channel covering the race. That bothered me, because we could have been at that race, and had we been there, I wouldn't have been in the crash with Jeremy.

Little did I know how unimportant my exasperation was about to become.

We were watching something on ESPN, and the "news crawl" at the bottom of the screen said something about the Charlotte race being interrupted or postponed because of a crash. That's all it said; there was no other information. Experience teaches you that any race postponed by something other than weather is often a bad sign.

When ESPN's *SportsCenter* began at 10:00, the lead story was from Charlotte, where there had been a tragedy. A car hit the wall coming out of turn four, shedding parts as it spun. As another car—the VisionAire car—passed through the scattered debris, it struck one of the wheels and sent it flying over the catch fence and into the stands. Three people were killed, with several more injured. The race was abandoned and never finished.

We watched the story in silence. It was a stark reminder of the perils of motorsports. I went to bed, suddenly questioning everything I wanted in life.

The Months of Fog

AT THE TIME OF THAT AWFUL CRASH IN CHARLOTTE, I WAS 16, and I had no idea how to process it. I didn't personally know any of those who'd been hurt or killed, so I worried that even saying something as simple as "it had a profound impact on me" could be seen as disrespectful. Some say that those on the autism spectrum lack empathy, but sometimes it's that we just can't easily express it. I know that in this instance, I was *full* of empathy.

The following week, I saw my psychiatrist. This period in my life was filled with such visits, and the diagnosis would change from month to month. Along with the varying diagnoses came the roulette wheel of medicines prescribed to me, which often had horrendous side effects.

On the very day of this particular appointment, I had learned that my ticket to the ill-fated Charlotte race was for the same section of grandstands, and very same *row*, hit directly by that flying wheel. That brought mortality into a bright light, and this was something I hadn't thought much about. If everyday things had occasionally been hard for me to process, trying imagining a subject as big as my mortality entering the equation.

Then I arrived at the doctor's office and was confronted with something that smashed every ounce of my processing ability. In the waiting room, I innocently picked up the latest copy of *Sports Illustrated*. That issue caused a lot of controversy because the editors chose to run a photo taken in the Charlotte grandstands after the crash; there was blood everywhere, and what were clearly bodies covered by sheets. I dropped the magazine and was frozen. Minutes later, when I sat with the doctor, I could not—*would not*—speak about what had happened. Honestly, I could not say much of anything.

I buried those emotions, but I questioned life, its meaning, and whether we had any choice in the events of our lives. That was a lot for my 16-year-old brain to make sense of. For a time I became withdrawn, uninterested in many aspects of life.

Working in the Alley

IF YOU'RE THINKING I HAVEN'T MENTIONED MUCH ABOUT my social activities in this period, it's because there weren't any. I liked being homeschooled, but one of its downsides was the utter lack of socialization. I was fully content with doing my schoolwork, watching the news, playing video games, and then repeating that the next day. My mom wanted to see me get out of the house, interacting with friends, but I found most people boring. Oh, I did have a few friends, but my interests were narrow; all I wanted to talk about and think about was racing.

Physical activity was one of the requirements for a passing grade with my homeschooling curriculum, and, sadly, racing didn't count. On a whim, my mom signed me up for a Wednesday-afternoon bowling league. I wasn't opposed to that, because I was pretty competitive and always loved watching bowling on TV as a kid.

Right off the bat, I did okay. My average score that first year was in the 140s, but by my second year I was up into the 170s. I was spending a lot of time at the bowling alley, and one day my dad asked the manager if there were any job openings. There was one, working Monday and Wednesday nights; when my Wednesday league game ended, my work shift began.

One problem was the thing I mentioned above: socialization. I still knew nothing about social cues and conventional social rules, or about the politics of the workplace. I was as naïve as naïve gets. I had a good excuse—I was on the autism spectrum—but no one knew that yet, including me.

I was given a work shirt that meant I was officially a staff member of Sunset Lanes. I'm sure I wore the shirt with more pride than anyone ever had. All I knew about work was what I learned in racing, where I always gave 100 percent. It was no different at the bowling alley.

So, there I was, working my first real job at the monstrous wage of $5.15 per hour. While the race track was glamorous work in my eyes, the bowling alley certainly was not. My duties included washing ashtrays, taking out the trash, cleaning tables, and answering phones if the night manager wasn't there.

On my first night, a Wednesday, the lady who normally worked Wednesdays was off, so the Monday staffer took her place. He was great with the customers, but thoroughly numb to every other aspect of his job. But he did a good job teaching me the basics, and I was soon an expert at throwing away beer bottles and retrieving ice buckets.

As the evening progressed, more bowlers started talking to *me*. This panicked me a bit; I didn't understand why they were talking to me. The conversations were all over the place as well. An entire team of ladies just wanted me to be there for them, and one of the men's teams blamed me for their scores. (Several weeks later, a man on that same team complained that the room was too warm, so he propped open the side doors of the building. This brought in a lot of humidity, which messed up the lane conditions. My fault once again, or so he said.)

I survived that first night, but I was tired. Working at a race track took a lot of energy, but this was a different kind of weary, more mental than physical. No, cleaning up after bowlers isn't a test of one's intelligence, but it did test my ability to be around people, some of whom may have had too much to drink, so instead of speaking normally, they yelled.

The wait until the following Monday was long. It was odd to suddenly have a job and then have several days off between shifts. Come Monday, the first guy I'd worked with told me to be careful on Wednesday because the woman who usually worked that night—"Carol the Terrible," he called her—would be back. He said, "Aaron, that woman doesn't like anyone, so be prepared for her to be mean towards you." I was ready for the worst.

Two days later, on Wednesday, I met Carol, and she didn't seem bad at all. Like the Monday guy, she showed a bit of apathy toward the job, but she was not apathetic toward drunks. She had no problem removing anyone who created a scene.

Carol said to me, "You're the shy type, right?" She was spot on, of course, but she would not accept my shyness toward her, which was good. It was a slow process, but the ice began to crack. We talked about certain bowlers and other bowling alleys and how the sport and its venues had changed over the years. I started to open up.

This was an important time in my life. I was finally able to have conversations, finally able to work with people. The self-image I had of being completely unlikeable was false.

I started looking forward to Wednesday nights. Heck, I might have paid the bowling alley just for the entertainment of working with Carol. This didn't go unnoticed by my co-workers, who jokingly wondered aloud if something funny was happening between us.

While my confidence went up, I still needed to learn the ways of the workplace. For Thanksgiving 1999, my dad and I planned to go to Oklahoma City. This would mean missing a Wednesday night shift. A couple of weeks before that, while bowling for fun on a Saturday, I mentioned to another lane attendant that I'd have to take that Wednesday off. He said that he was sure it would be no problem, and I figured that was that.

On that Wednesday, as we were passing through Joplin, Missouri, my dad's cell phone rang. It was Carol from the bowling alley, puzzled about why I hadn't come to work. Well, I was just as puzzled about why she was expecting me. I'd told the other guy that I'd be gone, so what was the problem? My dad later explained to me that a co-worker doesn't have the authority to grant time off. If I had to miss work,

I'd need to talk to someone at the supervisory level.

It wasn't the highest-paying first job—in fact, it was minimum wage—and the work was sometimes unpleasant. But the skills I learned at Sunset Lanes would help me down the road. That seems to be a common theme, doesn't it? We don't know what we're learning *while* learning it, and only later do we see the whole picture. This job, working in a casual environment with no real stress or deadline, started building my work persona. I was learning about others, but also learning about myself, cultivating the seeds for the next steps in my life.

Three Wide into Three

THE WINTER CAME AND WENT, AND Y2K WASN'T THE disaster it was predicted to be. After each shift at the bowling alley, I awaited the day that my racing career would progress into cars. I had no doubt that I was going to make it work.

As the 2000 karting season began, I told myself that I had to be even more aggressive than I had recently become. Being passive on the track isn't a winning strategy, so I started analyzing the other drivers. Racing isn't just about control of the vehicle; there's a heavy element of psychology that must be considered.

Who drives scared? Who is fearless? Who would have no remorse after slamming you off the track? To be a well-rounded racer, you must learn these things. Timid drivers will sometimes back off in side-by-side battles, even when they have the advantage going into the corner. I had been that type of driver, and others exploited it. Now it was my turn.

One driver who ran with the club had a chance of turning pro, but it didn't work out and for some reason he started driving timidly. He became hesitant when presented with passing opportunities, and I noticed that every time he was in three-wide situations, he'd hit the brakes and let both other karts go. In the first race of the year, I was running fifth, right on his tail, and he was just behind third. I got an amazing run out of the final corner, and as he went left to make a pass, he left a big hole in the middle. I jumped right into that gap. Three-wide through the middle is not an ideal place to be, but I *knew* both other drivers would lift, and they did. That pass was a two-for-one special. A week later, I pulled the same move on the same drivers.

Still, the results just weren't there for me at the start of 2000. Thirds and fourths were routine, but my craving to win was strong. And, in my defense, the pill draws often worked against me. It seemed I was always starting heat races in the middle of the lineup.

One week I drew the worst possible number. I'd be starting last in the first heat, and pole in heat two. In the first heat I moved up nicely, so a win or a second-place finish in heat two would put me on the pole for the feature. Starting beside me in that second heat was the defending class champion, Matt Riggs, who seemed to win no matter where he started. At the green he got the advantage, but I executed a nice cross-over move and we ran side-by-side through the next *seven* corners. It was amazing. It was *thrilling*. Our karts touched a couple of times, but innocently. Neither of us wanted to give way. The main-event pole was at stake.

In side-by-side racing on a road course, neither driver will have the preferred line in every corner, so they won't be running optimal lap times. This was happening with us, and I could hear the engine of the third-place kart behind me.

I was pretty sure it was a driver named Greg; he was fearless. If you went into a corner beside him, you could almost guarantee that he'd either hit you in the side or chop your nose off.

We had gone side-by-side for an entire lap. Now, out of turn two, I ran Matt a bit wide and thought I finally had a chance to get clear and perhaps win the race. But there was suddenly a sound to my left, and just before turning into turn three I briefly saw the yellow nose of Greg's kart. He was pulling *my* move, trying to pass Matt and me at the same time. I respected the audacity, but I wasn't going to give up, I wasn't going to show weakness.

That yellow nose had disappeared, so, thinking I was clear, I turned into the corner. Then I felt a thud, and I was sideways. I glanced left and was shocked to see the entire nose of Greg's yellow kart literally on my shoulder, but I felt nothing. My rear axle also hit Matt, and all three of us slid off the track. As we got into the grass, Greg's kart fell from my shoulder, and we all came to a stop. Matt quickly drove away while Greg and I both had damage that prevented us from continuing. Greg was able to limp his kart back to the pits, leaving me alone in the grass.

After the checkered flag, the race director walked over, and my dad was with him. I had never seen my dad this angry before; he was furious with the move Greg had pulled. He asked me about the moment we'd been three wide: "Did you know he was there?"

I said no, which wasn't *totally* true; I'd seen Greg's nose, and then I didn't. But my dad was already yelling at the race director. He wanted Greg disqualified and removed from the property; he thought the move showed a disregard for life and limb. I glanced away, because some of my moves, three wide up the middle, were as wild or wilder than anything Greg had done. The race director stood there and listened.

Seeing my dad fight for me like this was strange. As his yelling at the race director continued, I remembered the club rule that the driver is responsible for the crew's behavior at all times. I stepped between them, and said, "Dad, it's okay." Things started to simmer down.

Understanding love is difficult for many on the autism spectrum, including me. But while my dad's outburst was an odd way of showing it, I knew he was fighting for me out of love. Thankfully, the race director allowed him to vent. I didn't completely see why until later in my life, when I saw another racing father chirping at another race director. When I asked the race director why he hadn't thrown out the angry father, he replied, "When you become a dad, you'll understand. A dad will fight tooth and nail for his kid, and you've got to let him feel like he fought all he could." My dad fought as hard as he could because of his deep love for me.

From that day, I began to reassess my relatively new passion for racing three-wide. While one of the other two drivers might be timid, the remaining one might share my mindset of never backing down, and we might have a crash that could have been avoided.

Besides, I didn't want to be part of another incident that got my dad *that* fired up.

The Next Formula

RACING KARTS IN ST. LOUIS WAS FUN, BUT I WANTED TO move upward. My dad talked to many people about various racing schools, including the Derek Daly Academy, run by the retired driver who had raced both Formula 1 and IndyCars.

It was not inexpensive, but with a bit of sponsorship from my aunt, we booked a three-day November class in Las Vegas.

In the month leading up to the school, I was filled with anxiety. That was partly because one requirement for drivers was proficiency with a manual transmission, as well as the downshifting technique known as the heel-and-toe. In a nutshell, heel-and-toeing involves working all three pedals—gas, brake, clutch—at the same time, while also going fast and cornering. The trick to it is matching engine RPMs with wheel speed, otherwise the car might over-rev or wheel hop, at which point the rear brakes tend to lock up and spin the car. For someone unsure about the level of coordination between eyes, hands, and feet, it's daunting to even contemplate.

I spent hours in an empty parking lot behind the wheel of a junk BMW my dad got for this purpose. Just getting the car rolling and shifting from first to second gear was a challenge. Why, oh why, had all those racing games I played allowed an automatic-transmission option?

Eventually, I was able to make this ancient BMW move like it had in its youth. My soul soared anytime the car did what I asked. Then I'd try again and feel the rude defeat of stalling.

Ready or not, November came, and we landed in Las Vegas. As always, I was putting too much pressure on myself and turning this class into a make-or-break event in my life. What if I couldn't shift gears? What if I had zero car control with a formula-style, open-wheel machine?

Much of the first day was spent in the classroom. We were told how to climb into the cockpit, buckle in, and start the cars, and how *not* to accidentally trigger the onboard fire-suppression system. This was all necessary, but it felt as if the day dragged on. That was my fault; I was just so eager to get behind the wheel and feel the cornering forces.

Jeff Shafer, the instructor, did a great job in the classroom. I spent a lot of time looking at the diagram that explained the process of heel-and-toeing: First, brake for the corner; then, clutch in; next, position the right foot so the toes control the braking and the heel—or sometimes the side of the right foot—can blip the throttle; then, downshift, and let the clutch out. If you're going down more than one gear, as you often must, put the clutch back in, blip the throttle, downshift, let the clutch out, and repeat as necessary.

Oh, and do all this while decelerating from 100 miles per hour or more, while focusing hard on the proper line for the corner that's just ahead and getting closer.

Classroom time ended and the cars awaited, all lined up pretty in the parking lot. Getting into the Formula Ford was a thrill; I thought back a few years to being allowed to sit in Jonathan Byrd's IndyCar. Now here I was, in Vegas again, with a car assigned to me. If I could only shift gears, there might be more race cars in my future. But once the helmet went on and it was time to make the car move, there was the thud of a stall. Or two. Okay, three.

Before they let us onto the road course outside Las Vegas Motor Speedway, they wanted us to get fully familiar with the car's feel. Using traffic cones, they laid out a small oval in an empty parking lot. Jeff said, "These oval laps will not be timed. Speed doesn't matter."

Despite that, I was thinking about running hard around that oval … right up to the point when I was rolling around in second gear and floored the throttle. Even though this car had only 135 horsepower, the acceleration was unlike anything I had ever felt. It almost *hurt*; my sensory alarms went off at full blast. I remember saying aloud, "How does anyone do this?"

As I turned left into the corner, I was shoved over to the right side of the cockpit. That car flung me around as easily as a cat slaps a toy off a table. It was thrilling, but it was not *fun*. I could see it becoming fun, but that would only happen once I had a better feel for the car.

I wasn't accustomed to having to use all my chest muscles

just to breathe. And while I was thinking about breathing, I missed the braking zone for the corner and ran wide. I kept it within the cones, but I still had too much speed, so I jumped off the gas. That's when I recalled something else Jeff Shafer said: that driving a race car is about balancing weight. Get on the gas, and the weight transfers to the rear; back off, and the weight shifts forward; jump off the throttle too abruptly, and the back end gets so light that the car will want to swap ends. Right now, my car was threatening to do just that, but without hesitation or thought I gave it some throttle, applied some counter-steer, and prevented the spin. Okay, *now* this was fun.

That whole first afternoon was about getting acclimated to the forces, and being reminded how slow the human brain is. We were now in tuned BMW Z3s, running down a straight stretch of three-lane road. We'd come to a sensor that would activate lights above the three lanes; two lights would glow red, and the third would be green, and we'd have to move to the green lane. Sometimes all three lights would turn red, in which case we'd have to come to a complete stop. We were only driving at 45 MPH, but it was a real test of reactions and reflexes.

On the second day, we got to see the road course in the Formula Fords. It was a nine-turn layout, 1.9 miles around. It may not have been a fast-flowing track like Silverstone, or Watkins Glen, or Spa in Belgium, but it was a great course for learning. Speeds topped 100 MPH, and the sweeping right-hand turn six could be taken flat out.

Before we were unleashed to find our own pace, we had a lead/follow session in which we'd follow the instructor for a few laps. During this session, I tried the heel-and-toe, and it was just not working. I felt bad for the students behind me, who must have been puzzled about why my car lurched around in the braking zone and why there'd be times when it just wouldn't accelerate. As odd as it may have been for them, it was worse for me; I'd be wondering which gear I was in, only to discover that I was in neutral.

As I mentioned, my aunt had helped make this lesson possible, but there was still a budget to stay within. Any damage to a car was the responsibility of the student. Jeff had run through some of the ways we might hurt a car, and the list included colliding with wildlife big enough to wreck the front end. I did see three dogs wandering around, but thankfully no animals or cars were harmed that lap. Also, the dirt to either side of the track was full of rocks, so dropping a wheel off the track could kick a stone up into the engine compartment and knock off a timing belt. I'm not a mechanic, but I understood immediately that rocks meant repair bills.

On the back straightaway, I looked quickly at the car's display screen. It read: 105 MPH. And here came turn six, that flat-out sweeper. I was committed.

Inside turn six, my dad was sitting in a van with one of the instructors. I came into the corner flat out, but halfway through it my foot lifted off of the accelerator. Remember that whole bit about the weight transfer you get when you jump out of the throttle? At 100 MPH on a long corner, knowing that you've got more fast cars behind you, it's a great big deal.

The instructor in the van saw smoke come off my tires, indicating that I was sideways, and quickly said to my dad, "He's gone."

But I wasn't. I turned the wheel to the right in a manner that wasn't forceful, but gentle, and I eased back onto the throttle. The car transformed from angry, sliding beast to peaceful, happy race car doing what I wanted it to do. The instructor told my dad, "That's impressive. No one saves a car that far gone."

By the end of that day, my lap times had me in the top five out of a dozen students. Some in the top five had previous full-size car and/or formula-car experience; I'd never driven anything but a slow, four-cycle kart. And even though this wasn't a competition, I'm sure the competitive streak in all of us had us chasing lap times.

The final day was all track time. Riding there with my dad, I couldn't wait to feel the g-forces again. It was a stark contrast to that first day; the same forces that scared me then were something I now craved. I was acclimated to them, and I could feel the car. Getting out of the rental car at the track I whispered to myself, "Once again, I step out into heaven."

For day three, each car was equipped with data-acquisition gear recording everything from speeds and RPMs to throttle and brake inputs. Our laps would be compared to the instructor's, and that was a challenge. Jeff Shafer had been a winner in the USF2000 series, and also raced Formula Atlantics in the U.S. as well as Formula Palmer Audi in England. If I could get close to his time, I'd be thrilled.

Shifting was still a challenge; I had given up on learning the heel-and-toe downshift. But I had confidence in my car-control skills, particularly catching the car when it had wheelspin exiting the turns. The data would show that the RPMs had spiked, but my timing was right. In our debrief sessions, Jeff would comment that he had no idea how I maintained control.

The sun was getting low in the sky, and the final session was at hand. I was second quick, but I wanted to be the fastest. Even the potential damage costs now seemed irrelevant to the satisfaction that would come from being the quickest student, although I'm sure my dad's and aunt's bank accounts would've disagreed with that. I set out of the pits on a mission. And, yes, a part of me was thinking, "What if this is it? Racing is expensive. This could be my last time in a race car, the closest I ever get to glory in motorsports. Get after it!" And get after it I did.

On just my second lap, I approached turn six having decided to go through it flat out. I'd been breathing the throttle on entry and just cruising through, but that was leaving speed on the table. Approaching the corner at 106 MPH, I held my breath, turned in, and kept the pedal down. At the exit, my car drifted dangerously close to the edge of the track, but I stayed on the pavement stuff and screamed in elation. I'd done it. Then I slammed the brakes for turn seven, and focused on the rest of that lap.

When the checkered flag flew on the session, I drove slowly back to the pits. I was in tears. This school experience was better than I could've imagined. The g-forces were amazing, and learning to translate those sensations into how the car was behaving came naturally. In the debriefs I had a difficult time describing to Jeff what I was doing in the cockpit, and I think that's because it all came naturally and subconsciously.

Back in the classroom, the final data sheets were printed. My dad was with me when Jeff handed me my sheet and said I'd been one of the fastest students they had. He then cautioned, "If you ever test with a team, when it's over they'll compare you to Ayrton Senna, Alex Zanardi, or Michael Schumacher. They'll want you to feel good, and want you to believe that they'll do all they can to make your career happen. This isn't always true. They want your business and your money."

My dad then said, "So, does Aaron have it?" By "it," he meant the skill to make it in racing.

"Well, you've got to be careful," said Jeff. "I won in USF2000, so I had it and have it, but didn't make it."

My dad said again, "Does he have it?"

Jeff ended by saying, "If he gets a ride, he has it."

I think my dad was happy with that. He now knew that it wasn't just his desire to see me do well. It was my desire, too, my desire to do well. I knew I had "it" the first time I went sliding through turn six and didn't spin. The question was, what could I do with it?

Striking Out

RETURNING TO MY BOWLING-ALLEY JOB WAS DIFFICULT after my amazing experience in Las Vegas. There had been a change in staff, and one of the new night-shift managers was always on me to "talk more." I still couldn't force myself to converse just to make small talk. Working with him became more and more difficult, because I feared being reminded that I was unable to socialize. I couldn't understand why it was more important to chat than it was to keep the lanes clean and complete the other tasks in front of me. I went to work to *work*, not to feel like I was back in school, being chastised for not talking. The situation was wearing on me. I had been there over a year, and given the extra pressure I was feeling, I decided that I wanted a raise. I had started at $5.15 per hour, and that's where I still was.

I had just started a second part-time job, working for a video-duplicator service. I'd joined them right before I went to Vegas. It was the most monotonous work possible: For eight hours, I'd place 64 VHS tapes in VCRs, take out the 64 VHS tapes after they'd been copied, and put in 64 more. Then I'd label and box up the finished tapes. It paid $7.00 per hour, another reason for me to want a raise at the bowling alley. Besides, it would be a validation, a sign that I was doing a good job. The bowling-alley work was simple, but I did it with full gusto.

One night the bowling alley's owners were in town— they were from Florida—and I figured that this was my chance. I'm not sure why I thought I'd be able to talk bluntly to the owners, since I couldn't talk to the manager, but that was my intention.

During my shift, I kept walking by the owners, planning to say something, but words eluded me. I was hoping—no, praying—that the owner would see me and say, "Oh, hello, Aaron. I think you'd like a raise. No problem!"

I didn't understand this at the time, but I was again operating under that "theory of mind" practice that says, "I *think*, therefore you should *know*." I wanted this raise, and could not understand why the manager or the owners couldn't see that and make it happen. Just a nickel-an-hour raise, or acknowledgement of any sort, would've made me happy. I needed to feel like I was worth something to them, and having them "ignore" my silent wishes confused me.

I went through a second night of being "ignored" as I walked past them. Why couldn't they just make this easy? My frustration level was peaking. Earlier that day at the video duplicator, I asked if I could have more hours, and they said yes. Thinking about this, I made a snap decision to put in my two-weeks' notice at the bowling alley. That was it, just like that.

The inability to communicate can be difficult for those on the autism spectrum, and also difficult for those around us. They might not have any idea that we're frustrated over a situation not being addressed; they probably never saw whatever it was that we *wanted* addressed.

I didn't know it at the time, but this failure to communicate can leave behind crates full of sadness and loneliness.

Duplicating the Days

IN EARLY 2001, I WAS LOOKING AHEAD TO THE KART SEASON and realized that I wasn't nearly as excited as I had been in other years. I kept thinking back to the thrill of turn six in Las Vegas, or the precision it took to get onto the straightaways without spinning the rear tires. If I went back to that class, could I become their fastest student ever? Those things dominated my thoughts.

Also, I had learned that my karting division was going to have a low number of entries, and that bothered me. A top-five finish isn't exciting when there's only six or seven karts.

At work, I appreciated the sameness of each day. That's another quirk of many on the autism spectrum: We like repetition. But I did think it would be fun to have some sort of challenge now and then. If the VHS tape you're duplicating is, say, 44 minutes long, you can't shave off seconds—or tenths of a second—like you can when you're racing.

The idle time between duplicating, labeling, and boxing left me way too much time to think. For example, I now knew the thrill of driving at 100 miles per hour. What would 110 feel like? What would a three-wide pass be like in a race car, rather than a kart? I no longer had to imagine the colors, feelings, and smells of a real race car; I'd felt and seen all that. Pretty soon I was going to know what it was like to flash across a finish line first, with the checkered flag soaring above me. Yes, right after these 64 VHS tapes get the labeling treatment.

The months at the video facility passed slowly, but I was diligent, on time, and proficient at all I did there. As at the bowling alley, I had no idea if the owners thought I was doing a good job. One of the things I see now is that it would've helped me if jobs had scoreboards, like in sports, or grades, like in school. It would have been a way for people to know, without me telling them, that I was a good employee.

A storm rolled through St. Louis in the middle of a night in July. It knocked out the power, which deactivated my alarm clock, and I overslept. My eyes opened to a flashing 12:00 display on the digital clock. I looked out the curtains and saw daylight. I rushed getting ready and drove too fast to work, where I was 90 minutes late. I had never been late to any job, ever.

Everyone knew about the storm; there were limbs and powerlines down everywhere. I wasn't expecting any backlash from the owners, because the power failure was so easy to explain. I'm sure people showed up late for work all over St. Louis that morning. It wasn't a lack of effort, or laziness on my part; I had simply not been awakened by my dead alarm clock.

I'd been there about an hour, and things were running slightly behind. The owner's wife walked in and said, "Aaron, we need employees who are responsible, and you were not. We are behind today because of you, and this is unacceptable."

She walked away without another word. I was frozen. I had a 100 percent exceptional record on all the work I'd done there, and now, because of something Mother Nature had done, I was being spoken to as if I were a bratty teenager who needed discipline.

I didn't know how to react. I lacked the ability to put it into words and say something. As the seconds slowly ticked by, the beating of my heart grew more intense. A fury I didn't recognize surfaced; I'm sure it was boosted by my confusion over what it took to be on the good side of the scoreboard of life.

Slowly, I stood up. My breathing was labored, like I had a horse stepping on my chest. I looked straight ahead, unable to move. Then my anger subsided, replaced by a dark sadness. I had failed. That's all I knew. Maybe it was unfair, but it was still a failure.

I left the VHS room, went to see the owner, and said, "I can't work here anymore."

He said something, but to me it was like trying to overhear a conversation taking place in the phone booth on the other side of the room when you've already got two people talking right in your face. Whatever he had to say, it didn't matter. I left there broken and defeated.

Once again, my inability to communicate, or to understand the communication of others, meant the end of something good.

An Unexpected Skill at a Job

DEFEATED OR NOT, I HAD TO FIND ANOTHER JOB. AT THE time, I had a girlfriend named Emily, and she suggested I apply at a video game store at the local mall. After all, gaming was something I knew. I protested, because this job would require speaking to lots of people. My other jobs had minimal-to-no customer interaction, but a video game store would be totally different. This was a daunting idea. But with a push from Emily, I picked up an application and turned it in the next day.

A week went by, and the phone never rang. Emily suggested that I call the store, but using the phone was another thing I tried to avoid at all costs, so I drove to the store. I had not met the manager when I applied, but he happened to be working when I showed up. He asked me if I wanted to be interviewed for a position that had just opened up. I wasn't prepared, and I had never been formally interviewed, but I agreed, and the following 10 minutes seemed to me like the grandest of interview failures.

Job interviewing is one more thing that can be difficult for those on the spectrum. In fact, it can be infuriating because we know the subject, and we understand the work, but answering questions on the fly can be a tricky issue because of the amount of material we're processing. Here's an example: The store manager said, "So, looking at your application, it says here you are the chief starter for the St. Louis Karting Association? Does this mean you have management experience?" Management experience? Okay, this was tricky. I was managing the action on the race track, but I was not managing workers ...

That took about 30 seconds of processing, only for me to utter, "I ... I don't know?"

Yes, my answer took the form of a question, like something you'd hear on *Jeopardy!*

Next, he asked, "You worked at a bowling alley, so do you have sales experience?" Oh goodness, this was another difficult question. I did ring up sales, but there wasn't the "upselling" at the bowling alley that there would be at the video game store, where magazine subscriptions and other things were on offer.

Again, it took some time for me to issue basically the same answer: "I think ... I don't know."

My actual memory of the interview ends there, but I know it went on in this savage fashion for another eight minutes or so. It was awful. Leaving the mall, I could not possibly have felt like a bigger failure. These were easy questions, and I knew the answers, but my processing let me unable to respond in a timely or coherent manner. Why? That night I tossed and turned in anger that was almost a rage, wondering: What is *wrong* with me?

Yet the next morning the phone rang, it was the manager, asking if I could start work at 1:00 p.m. that very day. An awkward dozen or so seconds passed, and I said, "Yeah, sure ... I ... I can do that."

The mall on a Tuesday afternoon was an empty place. It was just the manager and I in the store, which presented a great way to learn the job without pressure. He took me into the back room and showed me his sales board. Ah, hadn't I just recently wished that workplaces had scoreboards, ways to be graded? The sales board had rows of names, and columns for subscriptions, game reservations, and MSTs, or multiple sales transactions. Just looking at it, and not yet understanding any of it, I wanted to be the best.

Even though the socializing aspect of the job seemed daunting, I had sort of been practicing for this job my entire life. See, I had played an enormous amount of Monopoly games. In Monopoly, it's all about trading and the way to win is to convince the person you're trading with that the trade is good for them even if it isn't. You've got to be confident and show no cracks. And when my first customer at the video game store was ready to check out, I upsold them to a magazine subscription. The manager couldn't believe it.

Quickly, I became the region's number one salesperson, by percentage. I wasn't working many days, but when I did, our sales board lit up.

I wish this was the end of that story, that all went well because I knew how to sell, that I'd found the job I was meant to do, but life isn't that easy.

My co-workers knew I was capable of conversation, because they saw me interact with customers. Imagine the slickest used-car salesman, and that was me in this environment. Slick, smooth, empathetic, whatever it took. However, once the customer left the store, I shut down. It was as if my brain were some sort of artificial-intelligence program that only switched on when a customer walked in. Showtime began when they broke the invisible plane separating our store from the rest of the mall.

This led to some confusion. Other employees tried to socialize with me, talking of music, movies, food, celebrities, and so on. I knew nothing about any of it. Sometimes when they attempted to make this friendly small talk, I would walk off to start alphabetizing a section of the store. I understand now I probably seemed as rude as one could be, teetering on the edge of downright snobbish. Did I think I was better than them? On the sales board, yes, I was absolutely better. But as a person? I most certainly did not feel that way.

I was confused by the fact that some of my co-workers never actually worked, instead conversing with other workers or with their boyfriends and girlfriends who came into the store. They couldn't or wouldn't be bothered with trying to better the store's sales record.

It should have been so simple: We had jobs, we got paid more than the minimum wage, and the bosses were fair, yet these employees didn't seem to be interested in working. Why did things have to be so difficult? Why did every job have a political or social side to it? Why should it matter that I couldn't hold a conversation with them unless it involved better sales tactics or more efficient ways to alphabetize? I loved those topics, so why didn't they?

The Chain of Command

THE THREE KEY AREAS OF INTEREST ON THE SALES BOARD at the video game store—magazine subscriptions, game reservations, and Multiple Sales Transactions—were established well before I was hired there, but that didn't mean that I didn't have my own thoughts about them. For example, reserving a new game cost $10.00, which would later be applied toward the actual purchase price of, say, $59.00. That was easily understood, and it made perfect sense to me until a competing store chain opened a location in the very same mall and offered $5.00 reservations for the same types of games. I could tell from the drop in reservations at our store that their lower reservation price was impacting us, and I mentioned that to the manager.

He disagreed, taking the viewpoint that no matter what the reservation price, the customer would still be paying the same price for the game.

"Whether it's $5 now, or $10 now, the end price of $59.00 is the same," he said.

That was true, of course, but the customer would probably feel like it's easier to lay down five bucks for a deposit, rather than twice that amount. I pointed out that our having fewer reservations backed up my theory. The manager countered by saying, "Well, of course the reservations are going to be down. Even if they're down by 50 percent, it's because there are now two competing stores at the same location."

Again, I had a different view. My own reservation numbers were down 75 percent, which told me that the 50 percent "competing stores" theory was wrong. We were losing business.

Perhaps I shouldn't have put as much thought into this as I did. After all, this was an entry-level job, and although the pay was slightly higher than minimum wage, it was not anything exceptional. Why would I care so much? The employee turnover rate was extremely high, which told me that most employees didn't care too much about working there. Well, when I do something, I'm going to do it to the fullest of my abilities. It's either all-in or all-out, and I treated every job as an all-in thing. In this specific instance, I was proud of my high sales numbers even though there was no bonus or reward on offer. I had reached number one in the region, and I wanted to *stay* number one.

I continued to lobby the manager for some sort of change, and at some point, he said that if I felt so strongly about this, there was a feature in the sales terminal's computer to email the corporate headquarters. So when my work was caught up and I had a few quiet minutes, I accessed the sales terminal, found the email feature, and began to put down my thoughts.

Explaining my case was easy. I used a little bit of humor to keep things light, but I made it clear that I was certain the reservation price was costing us business. When I was happy with the case I'd laid out, I hit the "send" button.

The following week, I was clocking in and the manager called me over. He said that he'd only been joking when he suggested that I contact the corporate office, and that the people there "did not appreciate" my email. He also criticized the fact that I'd used humor, saying "That email goes straight to the CEO!" He ended by suggesting that I "never use that email system again."

But, as he was walking away, he added, "Oh, and reservations are now $5."

Mission accomplished!

Actually, it was even better than that; the people at headquarters ultimately lowered the reservation price for all outlets operating with a competing store nearby.

As with most other things, I tried to look for a lesson in all of this. Up until that time, the chain of command within a company did not mean much to me. Yes, there had been that time at the bowling alley when I learned that I could only clear a day off with a supervisor, but that was not quite as serious as this. The email incident showed me that "going rogue" and trying to solve a problem on my own was not a good strategy. There are times when even if you're right, you're wrong, and this was one of them. I'd been right about the $5 reservation fee, but wrong in the way I brought up the subject with the big bosses.

Up to that point in my life, I thought it was fine to supersede any chain of command if I knew I was right. I've heard similar things from other individuals on the autism spectrum who ran into issues in the workplace; they were convinced that what they were doing was right, so they did not follow the proper steps.

What's the balance? Well, there are times when bypassing the chain of command is the correct play, but most of the time it isn't. Learning this dance can be difficult. In the case of the video-game reservation price, I attained my goal and helped our store stay competitive, which of course was good. But what if the store manager had fired me for bypassing him in the chain of command? Would I ever have spoken up ever again, there or in some other job?

For many of us on the spectrum, the chain-of-command concept is complicated by the fact that we put so much into the work, and we are easily frustrated when others don't have the same passion. Because of that, when we see something wrong, we'll try to solve it and pursue every avenue to make that happen, so if the chain of command is not clear, we might overstep without meaning to.

Some bosses might find that annoying. But shrouded in that potential annoyance is an employee with a level of dedication most employers should be pining for.

All's Well Until
Loss Prevention Comes In

THE MANAGER AND I BUILT UP A RAPPORT LIKE THE ONE I'd had with Carol at the bowling alley. It didn't happen overnight, but if it was just the manager and me, I was open and talkative. We even had deep philosophical conversations about the meanings of life and hope. We also had many friendly competitions; he'd attempt to outdo me on sales within specific time frames, but my winning record against him was extremely high.

In March of 2002, our store once again had the highest numbers in the district. When the manager let me know this, he said, "Aaron, when I hired you, I never could've seen you actually talking to people so smoothly."

Then came the next day.

It started when a man I recognized came into the store. A few months earlier, the assistant manager and I were working in the back room when this same man cracked open the door and stared at us. The assistant manager recognized him as the company's director of loss prevention for our region, so he was going to let the man do whatever he needed to do. Minutes later, he walked by us with a new Nintendo GameCube. The assistant manager and I looked at each other, befuddled. "Go ask him what he's doing," the assistant manager told me.

I caught up to the man as he was walking out the door and into the parking lot. When I asked him what he was doing, he said that he'd bought the GameCube for his son.

"No, you didn't buy it," I said. "And you're the loss-prevention manager, so this is an odd game you're playing."

He didn't seem to appreciate this, and as we walked back into the store, he said that we had failed on many fronts. He also said that we should never chase a customer out of the store the way I did. Had this been a test of some kind? If it was, why had he given me the story about purchasing it? I asked him that, and he didn't answer.

So now the man was back, this time carrying a suitcase. He walked straight to the back room, and the manager went with him, leaving me to oversee the store. Another employee showed up for his shift, and the loss-prevention man called for him.

When the manager emerged, I asked him what was going on. He didn't answer or give any indication that he'd heard me at all. Then out came the other employee, who looked at me with a flushed face and said, "Good luck."

The man opened the door and signaled me to come in. He told me to sit against the far wall. There was another person already back there who must have arrived while I was busy with a customer. She was an assistant manager from another store.

I took a seat, smiling but apprehensive. The loss-prevention manager hovered over me; I felt uneasy. Then he sighed, sat down, and said, "Aaron, do you want to go to jail?"

Wait! Jail? For what? I was as confused as I'd been in the job interview that I'd done in these very same chairs.

I shook my head in disbelief. "No."

"Well, then," the man said, "would you like to explain what's going on?"

I said, "Going on with *what*?"

My hands were shaking in fear, my lungs worked to breathe, and the room felt so claustrophobic that it weighed me down.

He said, "Oh, you know …"

"No, I don't."

He said, "The massive theft ring that's going on here."

I'm sure I took a long time processing this. Remember, processing *anything* took extra time for me. I'd seen shady-looking people who appeared to be buying and returning games. Was that it? For a moment, I thought about a defective Xbox I'd bought and returned, with the manager's approval. Was that what he wanted to know about?

I'm sure I was too quiet for the loss-prevention man. He said, "Aaron, the theft ring. I know you're in on it."

This was like a bad episode of *Law and Order: Video Game Theft Division*. The questions came faster and faster, and the threats of jail piled up. The harder he pressed, the longer the pauses before my responses. He finally had enough of my answers and non-answers and sent me away. I went back to the safety of the sales floor … but it no longer felt safe. I was sure a SWAT team was going to storm in, looking for that defective Xbox.

An hour went by, and my fear was over the limit. Zombie-like, I walked to the back room. Without a word, I sat down and stared at the loss-prevention man. Tears ran down my face. Then, out of nowhere, and almost warmly, he asked, "Aaron, do you like to golf?"

What? He led off with jail, and now we're talking about golf. Without waiting for my answer, he said that he would much rather be on a golf course. Whatever mind trick this was, it worked: I mentioned the Xbox. He looked surprised and said that no, he was not there for a single Xbox that would've been repaired and back on the market with no loss to the store.

There was also a bit of talk about the questionable people who'd been returning things, but he didn't seem overly interested. He wished me happy golfing, and that was that.

Over the next month, the district manager cleaned house. I was one of only two employees that remained. But the joy of sales had ended. The new manager didn't like the sales board, so that was gone. My hard work didn't net me anything extra in terms of money or respect. The back room now represented misery and fear, and I could not handle that.

In early May of 2002, I said to the manager, "I can't be here anymore."

"I can't blame you," he said.

That was more than 20 years ago, and I can hear that conversation clearly even today.

The Summer of Speed

MY DAD HAD STARTED DOING THE ADVERTISING FOR THE Derek Daly Academy, and the deal included a trade-out for me to take their five-day course. The first three days were similar to the earlier course I'd taken but would get me reacclimated to the car and speed. Days four and five would be more advanced sessions in which I'd experience slick tires and setup changes making for a faster car. Before then, however, I had a trip planned. I was meeting with a race team.

A connection made through an instructor at the Derek Daly Academy led my dad to talk to a team based in Michigan. They competed in the Star Mazda series, where the cars were a step up in performance from the Formula Fords I had run at the Daly classes. I would meet the team at the SCCA June Sprints at the Road America track in Elkhart Lake, Wisconsin.

My dad was busy, so I was on this adventure alone. Outside of trips to Indianapolis, I'd never driven solo outside of the St. Louis metro area, but the ride went well. I recall thinking: *This is how it starts.* As I neared the track, I began to get nervous. I'd never spoken with these people. I had no idea what to say, or how to say it. This would either go well or be a disaster.

I had seen Road America on television, but checking out the four-mile track in person gave me a sense of just how big it was. A credential was waiting for me at the sign-in building, and there was no missing the team's huge tent in the paddock. Maybe it was my lost look, but the team principal, Fabio Castellani, walked up and said, "You must be Aaron."

The next two days were a whirlwind of learning the names of team members and watching the sessions of their drivers from various corners. On my final morning, I sat in one of the cars to get measured. Thanks to more backing from my aunt, I had a test coming up after the five-day Derek Daly Academy course. Now, sitting in the car, it started to all seem real.

After the measuring, Fabio asked me if I actually wanted to be behind the wheel. I must have looked puzzled, because he said, "You seem to be apprehensive and reserved. I don't know if that's good for a driver. You have to be bold!"

Flatly, I said, "I'll show you when I'm behind the wheel what I can do."

He smiled, and with a slight Italian accent he said, "I like that answer."

A few weeks later, my dad and I were back in Las Vegas, where the summer temperatures topped 100 degrees. Driving at speed, the still air became a hot blow-dryer aimed right into my eyes. The first three days of the school were tests of fortitude and hydration. I had my mind set on the final two days, with those setup changes and slick tires.

On the fourth day, on went the slicks. Jeff Shafer, the instructor, warned me that I was now dancing on a razor. Yes, the tires were faster, but at higher speeds it would be more difficult to save the car if I lost traction. I thought about the slides I had in turn six during my first class. If I did that again, I might end up a passenger spinning into the rocky gravel runoff area.

There were no other students doing the four or five-day classes, so I was alone on the track. This eliminated the pressure of matching my times against other drivers, but Jeff kept me focused. He said they were going to change the setup after my first run, without telling me what they did. It would be up to me to adjust to the new conditions, and to explain whether the car felt loose, tight, or any of the terms you've heard racers use.

But on my second run, the car felt no different. The car's on-board display showed lap times, and they were in line with what I'd run in the first session. In the pits, Jeff asked how the car felt. When I told him I hadn't felt any change, he tilted his head and asked, "You didn't feel the car fight you, and not want to turn? Okay, let's try something else then."

The sessions that followed were more of the same. The mechanics made changes, but they didn't impact my lap times, and I wasn't able to describe what the car had done.

On the fifth and final day, my lap times remained consistent no matter what setups Jeff threw at me. Before each session, Jeff would tell my dad, "*This* time he'll notice." But I never did. Then, after lunch, Jeff had the mechanics make the car as loose they could.

A loose car is a one whose tail end wants to slide; most drivers have felt that sensation on snowy roads. Jeff's latest adjustment, he figured, would make the car almost undrivable; I found out later that he predicted that I'd come into the pits on my second lap to say that I couldn't stand it. But behind the wheel, I felt the changes, adjusted my approach—subconsciously, which is why I was having a difficult time telling Jeff how things felt—and carried on. My lap times were my best of the day, by a tenth of a second. Jeff couldn't believe it. As I rolled back into the pits, he was shaking his head in amazement.

The conversation we had before leaving began the same as the one at the end of my earlier three-day class. My dad asked if I "had it," and Jeff was quicker with his answer this time: I was one of the three fastest students they'd ever had. But he added that while my ability to adjust my driving to different conditions was a good thing, there was also a downside; a driver needs to feel and *understand* the changing behavior of his car so the team can know what adjustments it needs to make during a race. Still, I left Las Vegas with a new level of confidence.

Just 10 days after getting home to St. Louis, my dad and I climbed into the van and headed north to GingerMan Raceway in Michigan for my test in the quicker Star Mazda car.

The morning of the test, I had nerves I hadn't felt before. There's a big difference between driving in a school setting and testing for a team. I was glad to learn that the Mazda drivetrain made downshifts easier. For slow corners, I wouldn't have to heel-and-toe my way from sixth gear to fifth to fourth to third to second; I could go straight from sixth to second.

To make sure I was comfortable with the car's controls, the team had me drive around the pit access road. The first time I put the throttle down, I couldn't believe the power. Whereas the first time standing on the gas in a Formula Ford had pushed *me* back, this car seemed to push all internal organs to the back of my body. It was incredible.

After 20 minutes circling the pits, it was time to get onto the track. This was a proper road course, 2.14 miles in length, with elevation changes, hard-braking zones, and a couple of interesting corners with tricky apexes. Fabio stressed that I learn the track before worrying about my times; to be sure I did that, he taped over the onboard readout of lap times.

After my first session, Fabio told me he was impressed, and that my speeds would have qualified me mid-pack for the previous weekend's SCCA regional race event. He remembered what I'd told him at Road America about being quiet; he liked that, because people might not expect much, and then my speed would catch them off guard.

In the second session, I got faster and flirted with the Star Mazda track record. I knew something was up when I pulled into the pits; my dad gave me two thumbs-up as Fabio just shook his head.

After lunch, Fabio disappeared, and a mechanic released me onto the track. This time there were other cars on the track, with more teams testing. By now I had access to the onboard lap timer, and while I basically matched what I had run earlier, I could go no quicker. I didn't bother to check my mirrors much, because I'd had the fastest car on the track, but on one particular lap I happened to take a peek. I saw a tiny flash of silver and blue quite a way behind me, and then it was gone in a cloud of brown dust. Fabio had hopped into a car to check me out up close, and despite having new tires he'd run off the track trying to match my pace.

Fabio said later that my times were better than he thought they'd be. And then came something that reminded me of Jeff Shafer's warning about team tests.

"Look, I've seen some amazing talents before," said Fabio, "but you are a natural. You had never seen this track or driven this car, and you'd have taken pole and fast lap for last weekend's race. I'd have to compare you to Kimi Raikkonen in your natural God-given talent. Because of this, I think we could easily come down on how much a season with us would cost."

The number he gave me was high, steeper than anything I could ever hope to secure. So, although the test went very well, and although I proved my level of natural talent to myself and to others, I also knew that it would take well over a half-million dollars to make that talent shine in a series, racing against other talented drivers. In a way, this was the closing of an era of my life, but I was unaware at the time that the winds of change were on the horizon.

Pen and Teller

MY SUMMER OF 2002 HAD BEEN PHENOMENAL—DRIVING proper race cars and handling them well gave me so much satisfaction—but now it was nearly over. The karting club's season was winding down, too. The shortage of entries made the events a bit bland; many of the races were essentially settled by the second or third lap. That made both driving and flagging less exciting.

As autumn approached, Emily convinced me that I ought to take some classes at St. Louis Community College Meramec. I didn't know what to take, nor did I feel any urgency to do this; after all, my racing career was sure to take off shortly. But with her push, I enrolled.

It was also time for another job. My dad had a good relationship with his banker, and it just so happened that this fellow had moved to another banking company whose local branch needed tellers. After a couple of conversations, I was hired. My weeks became full: classes three days a week, and, after training at another branch, four days a week at the bank.

I had no idea what to expect from working at a bank. The manager intended for me to work the drive-thru booth, but it was still under construction. Some of the other tellers told me I'd be miserable, saying that the booth was like an isolation chamber, and that I'd have no one to converse with. Obviously, they didn't know me very well yet.

I could see that the staff at this branch was like a family. The general manager was the mayor of the town, the operating manager knew everyone, the cordial loan-application lady could dip in and out of any conversation with ease, and the three tellers I worked with didn't know what silence was. It was almost like being part of a 1950s TV sitcom, with constant, smiling chatter; my character would have been the odd man out who's trying to understand the local customs. I did not know that world. I never became part of the family or the conversations, and I wondered, again: Was something amiss with me, or was it was all of them?

My college experience revolved around three courses: Mass Communication 101, Appreciation of Music, and College

Composition 101. Unlike my previous school experiences, I found these classes highly engaging and interesting. The college comp instructor, Mrs. Wilcox, encouraged me to write, and I enjoyed it. In fact, during dull periods in my isolation chamber at the bank, I'd write down in pen things I needed to type later.

Incidentally, those other tellers chose the right nickname for that drive-thru booth because I was definitely isolated in there. It was a cramped, fortified, 4x8-foot space with a safe, a cash drawer, a retractable drawer for exchanging things with customers, a radio, and a chair for me. That was it, and I loved it.

Much like I had at the video-game store, I challenged myself in whatever category I could; in this case, it was transactions per hour. Our branch had two drive-thru booths, and on busy days when the lines grew long, my goal was to beat the woman who worked in the other booth.

On slow days, I was often the only person she could talk with, so we would chat via the intercom system that worked only between the two booths, and it was odd to have a conversation at work without seeing the other person. She was a single mom, maybe 45 years old, with a deep, philosophical mind. She got me to open up more than most people could, and I trusted her. When my drawer came up $3,400 short one day, she helped me solve the mystery. Thankfully, it was a simple keystroke error, rather than actual money missing.

And I daydreamed a lot about racing. My dad and I were trying to make things happen; we had a few lines in the water, and there were some nibbles, but not the bite we hoped for.

As winter descended upon St. Louis, the college term was coming to an end, and with it came some interesting grades. I'd had an injury on campus that required a hospital visit, and Mrs. Wilcox deducted points for my absence, dropping my composition grade from an A to a B. In music appreciation, my final grade was 89.99; the thing that kept me from hitting 90, which was an A, was the first question asked by the professor on our first test of the year: "What is my name?" Well, I'm terrible with names, and I mistakenly combined his name, Stillman, with his secretary's name, and answered, "Stillwell." That was a silly reason, I thought, to take away an A grade.

I told myself that it didn't matter because I'd be racing next year, anyway.

At Christmas, everyone at the bank got everyone trinkets or mugs of some sort, which I thought was pretty nice. But that afternoon, the manager walked through the snow to my drive-thru booth and told me that a lot of the managers and higher-ups had taken notice of me, and that I had everyone else beat when it came to average transaction times with no errors. She said she was impressed and compared me to another employee who had started as a teller and climbed to the level of senior vice president. Then she handed me a $100 Target gift card.

I was in shock. My other jobs had taught me that some managers didn't care about effort or even quality of work, so being told that people had noticed me and my work meant a lot.

I found out not long ago that this manager passed away back in 2012. I almost wish I'd never learned of that, because I'd have preferred that my lasting memory was of her handing me that gift card, and my surprise at learning that hard work does matter.

The last day of 2002, New Year's Eve, was a working Tuesday at the bank, and it was a slow afternoon. I think I spent most of it talking over the intercom with the woman in the other drive-thru lane. She asked what I thought my 2003 would look like.

Full of confidence, I answered, "Next year? It's the year that will make me who I am. My racing career will take off like a rocket, and I'll be happy."

2003: A Life Odyssey and The Beginning of Who I Am Today

THE NEW YEAR COULDN'T HAVE STARTED OFF WITH MORE promise. Just 30 miles out of town lived a man who was launching a prepaid gas card company and had plans to run a team in what was then called the NASCAR Busch Series. I had driven only open wheel cars and had no experience with stock cars, but I solved that issue by taking a class with a school that used the USAC International Speedway, a three-quarter-mile oval in Lakeland, Florida. I was the fastest student they'd had, faster even than a driver who went on to do some NASCAR Cup Series racing. That satisfied the would-be team owner close to home, and a whole plan was crafted for me: training sessions, tests, Late Model races.

I thought: This is it! This dream of mine is coming true. But first there was a little trip in the snow. Literally.

I had decided against taking more classes, so I was working more hours at the bank. On a wintery January day, I had a string of transactions that depleted my stock of $20 bills. I filled out a vault request, standard procedure, and walked into the main building of the branch.

I picked up three stacks of $20 bills totaling $6,000 and walked out the door. The spot where the sidewalk met the parking lot was snow-covered and tricky, and I slipped. In an instant, my legs kicked out in front of me, and I was looking straight up at the sky. I landed hard on my back, and my head smacked the ground. I later learned that I was stunned to the point that I didn't react to the first people who tried speaking with me. My co-workers called 911.

Waiting for the ambulance, I lay on the cold ground, covered by a mountain of coats. No one wanted me to move, for fear of a neck injury, but they had to keep me warm. At some point, I got my bearings and quietly told the manager to reach into my pocket; I still had that $6,000 in cash. She took the money, I went to the hospital, and thankfully nothing was broken, although it was suggested that I probably had a slight concussion.

A couple of weeks later, when I returned to work, I was no longer assigned to drive-thru duty. I was now inside, working as a regular teller. It was only then that I realized how perfectly suited I was to that drive-thru job. Inside the branch, I had to get used to socializing again; I also had some anxiety tied to my fears of a robbery. It's like everyone indoors was dancing to a step I didn't know and music I couldn't hear. They all moved so freely, without thought or effort.

It was maddening, frustrating, and it showed in my work. As good as my performance numbers were at the drive-thru, they were just as bad inside the branch. I tried claiming that I didn't feel right yet after the fall. I knew it was more than that, although I wasn't sure what it was. In the end, the anxiety became too great, and I left the job.

Yes, I got a bit down about that. But then I'd start thinking: What was a bank-teller's position at $9 per hour compared to a promising racing career?

Empty Seats at Empty Tracks

THE PLAN HAD BEEN FOR THE NASCAR SEASON TO START and the prepaid gas card company team to find its footing. Then funding would get me into the seat at tracks in the North Carolina area for test sessions, coached by a former NASCAR Grand National champion. That driver was excited, or so I was told, and I awaited these trips south to start the dream. I grew hungrier with every passing day.

The season started, and February turned to March, turned to April. The owner had been highly communicative in January, but with each week he got more and more elusive. One day in April or May, I saw him mentioned on the TV news, and not for a good reason. The company and the race team folded shortly thereafter.

It was back to square one. To be that close to a dream—having been told to my face that a team wanted to invest in my talent, with a former champion coaching me—and then to have it all disappear left me as low as I'd ever been. Lots of people have similar letdowns in their lives, and they'll know the feeling I'm describing. And if you don't know the feeling, I sincerely hope you never have to experience it.

A Meeting in Carmel

THROUGH A FRIEND OF MY DAD, WE GOT CONNECTED WITH a man who was said to be an up-and-comer in the racing industry. He had a new concept for team ownership and a plan to become the next powerhouse operation in NASCAR. As it was explained to us, this team owner wanted to train and develop a driver, raising the driver up from the short tracks to the Cup series. They were looking for someone like me.

My dad and I drove up to meet with him at a Starbucks in Carmel, Indiana, north of Indianapolis. He showed us his business plan and used the phrase "due diligence" more times than I could count, which for some reason made me ill at ease.

The meeting went on for several hours. We talked about

the former NASCAR Grand National champ who would coach me; you guessed it, the same former champion who'd been connected with the previous non-deal. This would-be owner was amazed that this champion had already heard of me. He said that made this one of those "has to be" situations.

Sitting at a meeting with someone telling you that all your dreams are going to come true is … *surreal.* There was talk of starting me on a salary as soon as I was signed. Half of my brain was telling me to jump for joy, and the other half kept me sitting there, emotionless, fearing that my hope and elation would be repaid with loss and despair.

As the meeting concluded, the man said that he was impressed with my knowledge of racing, with the things my instructors had said, and with the fact that I'd be willing to move anywhere, go anywhere, and do whatever was needed. It's an easy attitude to come by when someone offers you all you want in life. As I said in a YouTube promo video, "This was Plan A. There is no Plan B."

—— Aaron Likens: Professional Driver ——

SEVERAL MONTHS WENT BY WITH THE WANNABE NASCAR owner claiming he was still doing "due diligence," and he told me to do the same. He wanted me to get more seat time in any type of car to stay sharp. My dad was still doing ads for the Derek Daly Academy, so he called Las Vegas to see if they could help make something happen. By coincidence, their month of October in 2003 was jam-packed with BMW corporate events, and they were looking to hire another instructor. They asked if I wanted to come out there and work for the month. Without hesitation, I said yes, ignoring the fact that I'd never lived away from home and also ignoring a job I'd started a month earlier at another video-game store. When I explained the situation, the people at the store were great; they said my job would be waiting when I came back. One week later, at 4:30 a.m., I hugged my dad, hopped into my car, and headed west on Interstate 70.

The open road beckoned, 1,600 miles of highway. I could finally call myself a professional; after all, I was going to be paid to drive a race car.

I've traveled the country many times since that trip in 2003, but I don't think anyone forgets his or her first extended trip away from home. I was all smiles for miles and miles. By coincidence, it was a NASCAR race weekend at Kansas Speedway, and I passed a backup of traffic at the off-ramp adjacent to the track. I smiled wider, with the hope that it wouldn't be long before those same people could see me racing there.

After an overnight stop in Colorado and another day at the wheel, I made it to Las Vegas Motor Speedway and connected with Jeff Shafer. Socially, I was unsure how to act, and I may have been overbearing in my efforts to help. Thankfully, the only two students at the school just then were a father and son who seemed to enjoy my racing knowledge, so no harm done.

From the track, I drove the 30 miles to Henderson, Nevada, and met the family I'd be staying with for the month. Yes, I had some nerves; I'd never been away from home for more than a week, and never without my parents. But this family made me feel welcome, as if I were one of their own. I've never forgotten their warmth. Strangely enough, the wife's name was Sunshine.

The next day I officially started at the Derek Daly Academy. For starters, I had to learn to operate the "skid car," a regular BMW sedan with four caster wheels, one at each corner, attached by a subframe. Using a control box, an instructor can raise either the front or rear end of the car, at which point that end of the car starts riding on the casters, reducing the BMW's traction. The instructor can simulate understeer by raising the front end and oversteer by lifting the rear. The point is to make the student more comfortable with a car that's sliding and heading wherever its momentum takes it. It can be scary at first, but I had a blast learning it, spinning the car countless times.

The staff also wanted me to be proficient at autocross, a timed event in a parking-lot course lined with cones. The car was a BMW Z3, and I picked things up pretty quickly.

I was in heaven just driving the cars and being in this environment, and getting paid $275 per day made everything sweeter. At the end of the first afternoon, they wanted me to drive the highly tuned BMW Z3 on the road course. It was a slightly different layout from the one I'd run in my earlier visits, and of course this front-engine sports car didn't handle like the Formula Fords I'd driven previously. I drove with some hesitancy. One of the instructors led me around with another Z3, but his lines really didn't help me. I rode with him for a while, and his style was much different than mine; he would let the car drift. I could catch a drifting car, but I couldn't *induce* a drift. He had me try, but each time I'd overcorrect the car and the sudden traction when the wheels stopped sliding threatened to snap our necks. It wasn't the end of the world, and my lap times would suffice, but I wasn't as comfortable as I'd been in the formula cars.

Over the next of couple of weeks, I endured some social misunderstandings; there was a miscommunication about where they wanted a BMW parked, and I'm sure I seemed aloof when I ignored the other instructors who tried to talk to me. The truth is, I was intimidated. I was already on the back foot when it came to all things social, and it didn't help that everyone had an intense personality. For me, the only response was to retreat and be quiet.

I have to say, they *tried* to socialize with me. They invited me to lunch, invited me to dinner, and I could not say yes. I'm 1,600 miles away from home, and here are people trying to be friendly, and instead I stuck to a routine of eating at the Petro Truck Stop outside the track, driving to Henderson, and going to bed. On off days, I'd drive down to Boulder City and golf. One man I met, 60 years old and retired, told me, "Aaron, always slow down. Life will get fast, and before you know it, you'll be me, playing golf with someone 40 years younger."

Each workday, I'd leave before sun-up and drive 40 minutes to the track. One morning I was feeling peeved that in all the time I'd been there, I'd done no instructing in the formula cars; I'd have loved even a single session in one of those things. As I got to the school's shop, I saw TV news vans in the parking lot. I walked in, and the mood was somber. The previous day, in a private test at the Indianapolis Motor Speedway, Tony Renna had crashed and was killed. Renna had been an instructor at the Derek Daly Academy, and some of my co-workers knew him as a friend. I marveled at what pros these guys were; Tony's death obviously impacted them, but once the students arrived that day, they put away their grief and did their jobs.

The next day, I had finished my skid-car duties and was watching the formula cars lap the road course. An instructor in the flagstand beckoned me; he had to use the restroom. He handed me a stopwatch and told me to wave the checkered flag when time expired. I waved it with enthusiasm, which, unfortunately, turned out not to be a good thing. Some of the other staffers liked my flair in the stand, and that was pretty much the end of my driving time at the Academy. Don't get me wrong, I loved waving the flags, and the pay was the same in the flagstand as it was in the cockpit. But I wanted to feel the rush of the wind and the g-forces in the corners.

As the month of October concluded, so too did their need for extra staff. At 3:00 a.m., I pulled out of Henderson to start my journey home. It was a day of bewilderment. What did my future hold? I enjoyed my time at the Derek Daly Academy, but would I be invited back? I knew I didn't gel with the staff. Once again, I didn't know the dance steps; I could not hear the music.

I stopped for the night in Limon, Colorado. In my memories, time freezes there; in my memories, it is the happiest of places. In Limon, I stayed at the Econo Lodge and ate at Fireside Junction; neither place was anything special, but they are special to me. I was still naïve as to why I didn't understand the dance the way others did. I would find out soon.

The next day, I completed my drive back to St. Louis. When I pulled up in front of the house, my dad waved my checkered flag in salute. I'll cherish that sight forever.

Diagnosis: Autism

NOT LONG AFTER I GOT HOME FROM LAS VEGAS, I FELL into a depression. The video-game store job was there for me, but I made no call. I wasn't capable of working. I wasn't capable of much that November. Why was I idle at home when others were out living their racing dreams? Why had the man from Carmel not called? Would I ever drive anything again?

It was not lost on my dad that there had been something wrong with me for my entire life. Well, "wrong" is a subjective term; maybe "amiss" or "different" would be more accurate. But there was *something*. I realized that, too, at the start of December.

I'd gone back to Lakeland, Florida, to drive a late model. I drove down by myself, and on my first night there I ate at a Denny's. Right there, in the Denny's parking lot, I looked out my windshield and saw three kids, maybe brothers, playing keep-away with a baseball cap. I happened to be on my cell phone, talking with my dad, but I stopped midsentence and froze. Once again, I was seeing this dance that I didn't understand. How were these people so free? There was no formal beginning nor end to this game, yet it was clear that they all understood the rules, knew how long to play, and knew how much was *too* much.

Watching those kids made me break down and cry, heaving so hard that I could have pulled a muscle. For the first time in my life, I *accepted* that I was different. My memory produced scenes from events in my life, working backwards from the mismatch of personalities with my fellow instructors in Las Vegas, to the workplace games and politics I'd encountered, to my many issues as a boy at school. Was it all because of this *difference* I didn't understand?

Unbeknownst to me, my stepmom, Mary, had been opening up a dialogue with my dad about the possibility that *something* was there. As fate would have it, a current issue of *Parade* magazine had a story about an individual who had been diagnosed with Asperger syndrome. He was amazing at multitasking, pinball, and memory recall, yet there were other areas where he just didn't fit in. Reading that magazine, my dad realized that he could just about interchange my name with the name of the person in the article. I wasn't defective, I wasn't broken; there was a name for what I had. It was Asperger's, part of the autism spectrum. My dad saw that.

When I got home from Lakeland, my dad said that he

wanted me to undergo an "assessment." This sounded no fun at all, especially when I learned I'd have to talk about my emotions. This, I wanted no part of. Writing these words, I can be open about things, but back then any question about my emotions would get you only an "I don't know" response. To cheat this system, I decided I'd write down everything I wanted to say aloud but couldn't.

I sat down at my computer, opened a new Word document, and typed: "I Wish …"

I was amazed at how many words were written. But the next day, at the assessment, the man in charge was having none of it. I kept saying, "The answer is in the document I gave you," but the assessment gauges behavior, so anything written would be of no value.

The assessment took three or four hours, and some parts were actually fun, but the parts dealing with emotions were not. When the assessment was complete, I had to see my doctor, which I did, alone, the week before Christmas.

I wasn't so sure about this doctor; I'd been with him before, and never knew what to think about him. He was in rare form, though, on this day. He stepped into the room, with the assessment in hand. He thumbed through it and made some grunting noises. After a dozen or so seconds, he flipped back to the front page and the summary and said, "You, there's no doubt about it, you've got Asperger's. I don't really know what to say. Good luck?"

I didn't know what this meant. Asperger's? I'd seen a couple of things on news shows like *20/20* and *Dateline*, but I never thought I'd be in the same category as the people they covered. Also, I had been diagnosed with so many things in my school days that I didn't put much stock in anything anymore.

But that evening I sat down at my computer, logged onto the Internet, and looked up this thing called Asperger's. I clicked the first page it gave me, and that's when fate struck.

The site I landed on was not, shall we say, medically accurate. But it listed some symptoms of Asperger's, and I matched up with a lot of them: "Uncomfortable in own skin" was one that stuck out, along with "socially awkward." Then came a line that shattered my world: "People with Asperger's will never have a job, will never have friends, and will never be happy."

My heart was still beating, but I felt dead inside. I thought about the struggles of the past year; I had gotten close, at times, to living my dream, and now I was being told that having a dream was pointless because failure was already a certainty. This blackened my heart. Looking at it logically, why put in any effort, *anywhere*, if the outcome is already decided? The collateral damage of this diagnosis was me sending a breakup text to my girlfriend on Christmas. She, too, had looked up this diagnosis on the internet, and got bad information that I was incapable of love. I asked her in the text if she still liked me. Yes, social awkwardness indeed.

To make matters worse, the very next week that would-be NASCAR team owner in Carmel said that, starting soon, I'd be getting paid to have a "lifestyle." That was the last we heard from him. Also, we met with a team that said they wanted to race a NASCAR Truck, an ARCA car, and a Late Model. They were looking for funding, and their figures seemed a bit funky. They were con artists, looking to make a quick buck.

Is it any wonder that I started believing all hope was lost?

I simply watched the days pass by. I didn't look forward to waking up in the morning, or the afternoon, for that matter. In my dreams, anything was still possible. Waking up brought only this notion that I was sentenced to life as a failure. I saw myself as nothing more than a waste.

In life, when you believe in what you're *not*, you very

well may forget who you *are*. I know because it happened to me. My talents, my experiences, my essence in life were lost.

I stayed this way all winter. My dad attempted to pull me out, but anything he suggested was met with a flat, emotionless "no."

The one thing I did not give up on was racing. I was still chief starter for the St. Louis Karting Association, and I took on more duties as the 2004 season approached. I did quit driving karts, but working in the sport—the idea of being at a race track—was a glimmer of light in a dark tunnel.

—— 2004: An Oasis in a Raging Storm ——

EVEN THOUGH RACING WAS A BRIGHT SPOT FOR ME, I WAS more apathetic than I'd ever been. In the late weeks of winter, I felt numb, defeated. I'd often not know what day it was. It's hard to describe the sensation of changing, almost in an instant, from knowing without a doubt that dreams will come true to believing that everything is impossible.

The local karting season was due to start in March, and I was asked if I wanted to direct and run the Saturday practices. I agreed, but I had a sense of apprehension; I'd never been the director of anything. Even as chief starter, overseeing start/ finish, I was carrying out procedures rather than directing things; I was an efficient messenger, but I was not the one dictating the messages. Now, though, I'd be setting the practice schedule, the times that the sessions would run, and more. At 21, this was an important building block.

Life is funny. I can see now—even if I couldn't see it then—that amidst all the turmoil I'd been feeling, I was also piling up skills and experiences that would help me on the next road.

One lesson I learned on my very first day of directing practices was this: Do not start a sentence with the words, "Nothing ever…"

The club had engaged a new EMT, a man named Roy, for the entire season. As the day progressed, he started asking me about racing procedures and what the average number of incidents per day was between a practice day and a race day. I said, "You'll have some crashes when we're racing, but nothing ever happens on a practice day." Well, with timing straight out of a scripted TV show, that very instant a kart failed to slow for the 170-degree radius first turn and instead went straight, which led him toward the pit entrance. On that entrance road, there was a tight 90-degree corner just before the pits, but this kart was not slowing down. Roy and I rotated our heads in unison, following that kart's every move, not believing what we were seeing.

Running flat out, he had no chance to make that last turn. His kart plowed through a closed gate; his helmet struck the padlock, and the driver was wrenched back by the blow. The kart traveled some distance before stopping against another fence. I grabbed the red flag and ran to block the pit entry to stop the session.

Once I was sure no other karts were coming with any speed, I hurried to the scene, preparing for the worst. But, like everyone, I was shocked and elated to find that the driver was awake, alert, and, almost miraculously, none the worse for wear.

That day gave Roy two lessons, and reinforced those same messages for me: First, do not put any weight in the notion that something "never ever happens" in a particular circumstance; second, even when things seem quiet and routine, as in a practice session, always remain alert. The calmest of days can turn critical in an instant.

The next couple of practice weekends came and went, and I proved to myself that I could handle this new leadership role. I wouldn't have admitted it at the time, but I took great pride in this. I'm sure there were many weekdays when I seemed blank or down, but directing these practice sessions and continuing my flagging duties proved an oasis for me.

———————— **A Secret Diagnosis** ————————

WITH THE ASPERGER'S DIAGNOSIS ON PAPER, I KNEW WHAT I had, and my family knew it, but I had no idea how to discuss it with others. Should I mention it at all? The Internet said that I'd achieve nothing; if someone knew I had this condition and found the same information online, would they also believe this about me? I remember having a first date with someone at about this time, and when I brought up my diagnosis, she said, "Asperger's? That's autism, right? That means you're incapable of love." She said this not as an opinion, or as a question, but as a fact. You know how people say that words can hurt? Well, that was an impalement.

At this same time, I started racing online. In just the first two days, I had so much fun that I wrote in my journal, "Who needs friends? I've got Xbox Live!" Truly, I was having the time of my life. People commented that I was a fast, clean racer. One note of interest was that although these games encourage interaction, and although I had a headset and microphone, I did not speak. Why would I want to? These people were competitors, not friends.

Just weeks after I started racing online, a new game debuted. It was called TOCA Race Driver 2, and I excelled at this game; in fact, it wasn't long before I was ranked number one in the world. Sadly, I suppose, I was a professional gamer before that skill could be monetized. I still wasn't speaking to the other players. My dad would say, "Aaron, you've raced with that Jason guy or that player named Naval for several days. Why don't you say hello?"

I'd say, "Why would I want to do that? One of them could be a serial killer. Besides, no one talks on here." That was a lie, and he knew it. He could overhear the voices from my headset.

My silence led to some funny moments. People began to speculate on my identity, and it was hilarious to hear. Some suggested that I was a 6-year-old prodigy. There was even a theory that I was Kimi Raikkonen, the Formula 1 World Champion from Finland, because I hadn't played on some weekends when the real Kimi was busy with F1 races. Eventually, I unmuted my mic and came clean. I even mentioned that I was on the autism spectrum, and that turned out to be a good thing. One of the other players had a child on the spectrum, and after we talked a bit, he mentioned that he owned a "driving experience," which is similar to a racing school but is more about letting non-racing motorsports enthusiasts feel the thrill that goes with driving a car. He had some dates set up at Pocono Raceway in Pennsylvania and said that I was welcome to come out and help. I said yes immediately. So much for my fear of online serial killers.

Much like my drive to Las Vegas, the trip to Pocono was freeing. I needed this; I needed to prove that I was capable of navigating life, and that the walls of our home were not the ends of my universe. It helped that when I disclosed my diagnosis to the other online racers, I was not met with scorn or confusion, and in the case of this man there was real understanding. We discussed autism with an air of normalcy; it was not something feared or looked down upon.

I met him and his family the day before I'd be helping

out at the track. This was one of the first open conversations I'd had about autism. Maybe I was disarmed because I was in a new environment, but I spoke in real-world terms, and not with my usual catastrophic outlook.

My duties at the track were unlike anything I'd ever done. My job was to finish buckling in the drivers, which involved leaning *way* into the window of a stock car and approaching belts and harnesses from a different angle; I usually had a hard enough time buckling my own five-point harness. Also, the scene on pit road was very dynamic, with cars coming and going and lots of people moving about. This was not my strong suit.

The owner of the driving experience was a bit concerned. I learned later that he called my dad and mentioned that I was like a puppy lost on a busy interstate. I can imagine his confusion; he'd seen me in my element, fast and full of confidence on Xbox, and I'd been able to express myself with his family, yet he saw only trepidation when I worked with people on pit lane.

The driving experience was only open for two days, and the time passed quickly. At the end of day two, I was shocked when the owner invited me to climb into one of the cars and run some laps. While these were basically NASCAR Cup cars, they did not reach the same speeds, but they were plenty fast on this 2.5-mile tri-oval. Pocono's first turn, at speed, was a new sensation for me; it was a reminder that I'd never been in a corner with that much banking.

On my next-to-last lap, I lived out an instruction I'd been giving people for two days: "Never turn the wheel right. If you feel the car sliding and you're losing control, just let it spin to the left. If you turn it right, you might go head-on into the wall." As I approached turn two at a good speed, rain drops appeared on the windshield and immediately increased; a steady rain had just blown in, and I was driving into it. I had slowed down with the first drops, but the slick tires had already lost traction, and the car started to skid. Instinctively, I turned the wheel right. But before the car hooked in that direction I was already steering back to the left. Luckily, my timing was just right. I didn't spin into the infield, and I didn't nose the car into the wall.

Well before dawn the next morning, I started my drive back to St. Louis. That's a 13-hour trip, so I had lots of time to reflect on the past six months. It was the start of May, and six months since I'd learned of this thing called Asperger's. This trip had shown that I could be happy; I enjoyed talking with this man's family, and I loved the chance to make laps at Pocono. Even driving on a lonely highway in the dark brought an eerie sense of satisfaction and joy. For the first time since my diagnosis, I allowed myself to feel … *hope*.

A Season's End

THE END OF THE RACING SEASON HAD ALWAYS BEEN DIFFICULT for me, but in 2004 it felt worse. My weekend routine was rather rigid; each day I headed to the track I'd listen to the same music in the same order, I'd stop at a 7-Eleven and get a Red Bull, then I'd stop at a Waffle House for breakfast. I'd much rather have had a routine racing cars somewhere, but this is what I had; it was my life, my world, my everything. And now, at least for the winter, it was coming to an end.

Roy the EMT and I reflected on the year that was, looking back on that first practice day when we'd met. Now, neither of us knew whether we'd be retained for the following season. Life had given me so many reasons not to be optimistic, and although I loved the smell of autumn and the trees were full of color, it felt as if my world, like the track, was getting ready to close down.

Sunday brought amazing weather. The air was cool, crisp, and clean, and the blue sky seemed to be making an extra effort to be even bluer. My routine stayed intact, but I was in tears as I paid at the Waffle House. All winter, my days would be filled with nothing but online racing. I loved the idea of competing for number-one status, but I knew that I belonged at a track. What if I wasn't invited back in 2005? The thought was overwhelming.

Catastrophic thinking is a common trait of those with Asperger's and on this day I was turning pro when it came to dire predictions. As I left the Waffle House, I wondered if I should just skip the day's racing and go home. If I did, I wouldn't have to go through the pain of waving my final checkered flag.

The fail-set mindset is one of the most difficult things about living with autism. It says that if failure is a guarantee, why try at all? Once it is triggered, motivation disappears. Picture yourself at a carnival: For $10, you can play a game whose prize is a colorful stuffed animal. You know the odds are against you, but the fact that you've got a chance convinces you to play. Now, imagine the attendant confiding in you that the game is rigged, and that your chance of winning is zero, zilch, nonexistent. You absolutely would not play. Let's modify that example a bit: What if you've already paid your $10 and had one attempt at winning before the attendant tells you that little secret. How many more attempts are you going to make? None. This is what life can be like for us on the spectrum. We've been told that parts of life are rigged, so why continue? And by sinking into this mindset, we help rig the rest of life against ourselves.

I sat at an intersection, full of doubt. If I turned left, I'd be home in minutes. If I turned right, I'd be on I-55, heading toward the karting track. I knew where I belonged. I turned right.

The day was smooth and without drama. I was able to do my job, although I was counting down the number of heats and features left in the season. Each one was like another tick on the time bomb I had constructed in my head.

I put a little extra pizzazz and a lot more passion into my last double-checkered, then started rolling up my flags. Someone asked if I wanted to stick around and help pick up trash, because the club always left the park clean. Usually, I'd be the first one out of the track; I wasn't one for small talk. But this time, I figured I might as well milk every second from this day. We walked the property until the sun was gone and the temperatures dropped. It was time to go.

I went back for my flags and headed for my car. And as I walked past the club president, he thanked me for my work and said, "See you next season!"

Next season. There would be a *next*, and that was all I needed in life.

Finding Kansas

I HAD JOINED TWO BOWLING LEAGUES, WHICH HELPED ME pass the weeks, as did my Xbox racing, but winter left me too much time for reflection. I looked back on social errors I'd made, and my rigidness in life, and cross-referenced all of that with the website that told me there was no hope. Each day, the shouting in my head got louder. How could it be that in the right environments I always proved to be extremely capable, yet I had read and been told that I had no chance? Was it really that black and white? All I wanted was for someone else to know of these thoughts, to *understand* them. I felt like a giant burden to anyone and everyone, but maybe if they understood, at least for a second, I'd feel free.

One night in February 2005, I remembered the "I Wish…" paper I'd written to avoid talking at my autism assessment. Although it was ignored in our discussions that day, it had given me relief. I went to the computer, opened a Word document, and I started writing about the first girl-friend I ever had. Four hours and 19 single-spaced pages later, I had … *something*.

It was 3:00 a.m. Everyone but me was asleep. I had created this small universe with words, but did I dare share it with anyone? What would they think? Was I wrong to express myself? I thought about emailing the document to my dad, but instead I printed it out. Hearing the printer go on and on, spitting out 19 pages, was a minor thrill; I had gathered a lot of thoughts on those pages, and I felt better having done it. I'd had all of that shouting inside my head, and these words were a way to make myself understood. I didn't have a book in mind; I simply wanted my parents to understand why I was the way I was.

I placed the 19 pages on the stove, where I knew my dad would see them in the morning. And as I walked down the stairs to my bedroom, I felt a familiar thrill. Yes, this was the same as those three-wide moments I'd felt in racing, living life at the absolute edge. I didn't know the simple act of writing could be so liberating. Now, having discovered this, I had *two* things to look forward to: racing and whatever I ended up writing next.

My work got a two-word review from my dad: "Not bad!"

So, I kept it up, discovering who I was and why I was, and writing what would ultimately become *Finding Kansas*.

— The Attempt at Producing What's Next —

WHILE I WAS THRILLED TO AGAIN BE FLAGGING FOR THE SLKA, the $150-per-weekend pay would not support me. My dad knew I needed something more, so he took a chance and called Lingner Group Productions in Indianapolis, which produced the IndyCar telecasts, including the Indy 500, for ABC. First, he asked me what I thought. I'd never considered that side of racing, TV production, but it sounded interesting.

I'm sure production companies get lots of cold calls from people wanting to break into television. But in the conversation, my dad learned the fellow on the other end of the line was an online Xbox racer, so he mentioned the screen name I used. Not only did this man know me, but he said, "I've never beat him!" Instantly, we had an appointment to meet two weeks later.

It was a cold, drab day when we drove to the Lingner office in Indianapolis. I knew their work; in addition to the IndyCar broadcasts, Lingner had also produced ESPN's "Thunder" series of USAC racing. We got an office tour from the man who "knew" me, and he thought I might fit into their intern program. It was too late to get onboard for the IndyCar opener in St. Pete, but he was hopeful I could be part of the month of May at Indianapolis.

The day had gone well, and at the end we met Terry Lingner, the owner, and a motorsports TV innovator. He struck me as an intense person. Right away, he asked a question that took me a bit to process: "What do you want to do in racing?" I mentioned my desire to drive, and he asked my age. He said, "Aaron, if you work for us, you may never under any circumstances talk to a team owner about a ride." Then he went full Simon Cowell *American Idol* on me and said, "You're 22. Time's running out. You need to either shit or get off the pot."

Those were the harshest words I'd ever heard on this

topic. Maybe I was naïve and still thought the driving career might work out, but no one had told me that perhaps it wouldn't.

I was a zombie after that. I don't remember how the rest of the day went. I hyper-focused on his words, and I hated them. But I wasn't angry at Terry. I was 22, and a 22-year-old driver should have already advanced beyond karting. He knew the industry. I was the one trying to convince myself that there was still a chance.

At the very end of April came bad news from the Lingner group. ABC had taken over the intern program, and it was now exclusively for handpicked college applicants. That might have been a godsend, and I'll tell you why.

Not long after that, on the opening day of practice for the 2005 Indy 500, I had a huge mass on my neck and a 104.5-degree fever. I went to the emergency room and was admitted. By now, I was almost delirious from the high fever and horrible pain. Believe it or not, the same doctor who'd told me "Good luck" after my Asperger syndrome diagnosis was on duty; he tried to discharge me, suggesting that the mass on my neck was "just a spider bite." My dad basically fired him, and another doctor quickly put me on intravenous antibiotics. It turned out that I had a severe infection—methicillin-resistant Staphylococcus aureus, or MRSA—at the base of my skull. MRSA is brutal. But here's the thing: Had I landed that internship with Lingner, I *know* I'd have gone to work, sick or otherwise, rather than risk losing the job. And had I done that, there's a real chance the infection could've spread, and could very well have ended my life.

Challenging Authority

MY ROLE WITH SLKA GOT MORE INVOLVED AT THE KART track as the season progressed. I flagged just two weeks after being discharged with the MRSA infection, despite a hole in my neck that our EMT, Roy, had to repack and re-bandage twice a day. You've heard stories of racers hiding injuries to keep doing what they do? Sometimes officials do that, too. Unless I was barred from working, I was going to be at the track.

Late in the 2005 season, I became race director for the shifter karts, the fastest type of go-kart. Our usual race director competed in shifter karts, so I would be the chief referee for that class.

The club started experiencing unexpected and immense growth. A new shop in town, PG Racing, was thriving; through their sales and more modern equipment, there was a karting boom in St. Louis. This made flagging a thrill, because the grids went from six–12 karts in some classes to fields of 16–24! On the next-to-last weekend, there was a great turnout of shifter karts and the top two in points were close. Driver Gary Shekell, who was also the club's two-cycle engine-tech director, needed a top-three finish to clinch the championship. Should his opponent win and Gary finish outside the top three, it would be tied. This was a critical race.

In racing there are rules, and outside of those dealing purely with technical matters, most have to do with safety. At club-level karting, safety infractions are often met with a draconian response. For example, the rule book stated that "any pass in a yellow-flag zone will be met with a black flag and a race disqualification." That rule is there for the safety of both drivers and officials who may be tending to on-track situations. It's a black-and-white rule, with no gray area. Early in the shifter-kart race, two karts ended up in the barrier, bringing out a yellow flag in that turn, and Gary passed another kart in this zone. It was a lapped kart, not one he was battling for position, but that didn't matter; he had passed a kart in a yellow-flag zone. It was as plain as day, so without hesitation I black-flagged him. Gary did not pull in, as required; instead, as he passed by on the next lap, he raised his hand in the universal gesture for: "What the hell?"

On the following lap, he slowed dramatically in front of the field, causing the pack to scatter, then pulled over and parked at my feet. This move itself would be a major infraction. Then he motioned me over to have a discussion. It's common to see baseball managers have on-field chat with umpires, but it isn't safe or proper to have a debate on a live track.

He kept waving me over, so when no karts were coming, I went to him. He said, "What did I do?" I told him that he'd passed under yellow. He didn't hear me, so, relying on my own sign language, I showed him the yellow flag and made a passing motion with my hand. He indicated that he didn't understand. The field was now close to the end of another lap, so I had to get him out of there. I put on my most serious face and motioned for him to get going. He hesitated but drove on and entered the pits.

There was a lengthy discussion after the race. I brought in the driver who'd been passed in that yellow zone and another witness to convey that Gary had, in fact, made the pass. In his defense, he may have made an honest mistake; he was adamant that he had seen no yellow flag, perhaps because he was so focused on getting around that slower kart. But black-flagging Gary was the right call. The penalty may have been a bit severe, but the rule was the rule.

All of this was complicated by an issue that had little to do with the actual racing: Had he locked up the championship—which he might have done without that black flag— Gary was not going to race the following weekend. He had made other plans. Now he had to change them.

The next week, I was getting ready to wave the checkered flag to end a shifter-kart practice session when I heard a corner worker's scream on the radio. I looked up the track and saw a kart flipping. I threw the red flag rather than the checkered. This was a serious crash, and it was Gary Shekell. The EMT rushed to the scene. An ambulance was called, then a helicopter.

This was critical, and in those tense moments I blamed myself. It was common knowledge that Gary wasn't going to run that race. My black flag and his disqualification forced him into it. I couldn't think myself out of the equation; my actions had led to Gary's crash. I was terribly concerned for him. He'd been racing with the club long before I ever showed up, and his brother was the first race director I raced and flagged under.

The next day we learned that he had suffered broken ribs and a collapsed lung, but that his injuries were not life-threatening. I breathed a heavy sigh of relief, happy that he was going to recover. My brain was weighed down by the gravity of the situation, but I accepted that my action was right. I didn't make the "pass under yellow" rule, and I didn't cause the next week's crash. I wish I could say that the thought of quitting never crossed my mind, but it had. A lot.

Racing is dangerous. We fool ourselves into thinking that if we do our jobs perfectly, whether driving or officiating, we can erase the danger, but it's there. And when it surfaces, you naturally wonder if it's worth it. But anytime I've had that thought, I've concluded that yes, it is.

Gary made a full recovery. In a strange twist of fate, our black-flag incident led to my next gig, the one that started my climb up the ladder, and Gary would be a coworker.

Becoming the Authority

AS THE CALENDAR SWITCHED TO 2006 THERE WAS TURMOIL within the kart club. The race director got fed up with the complainers that come with the territory and resigned. I thought about trying to step into that role, but here's the thing about being a race director: It's a no-win position. You will not be thanked for doing your job well, and when you have to issue penalties, however correctly, not everyone will be happy. The paddock will say that the race director is too strict, too lenient, too hot, too cold, too ugly, and causes disagreeable weather. True story: I actually heard a race director blamed, and not in jest, for the weather. Why would I want any part of that? Oh, and the race director has to conduct the drivers' meeting, which means speaking to a crowd. No thanks.

A month went by, and the position had not been filled. Meanwhile, Greg Yocom, the owner of PG Racing, was planning to start a regional karting series. I had never talked with him, but Gary worked for him, and the man took notice when I black-flagged the tech director. He needed a flagman for his series, and more, so he gave me a call.

I don't like talking on the phone, and never have, but I spoke with him. I was hesitant, because he had a lot of customers who raced, and I felt that in their eyes, my talking with him might compromise my objectivity at the kart track. I assume it's the Asperger's in me, but I've always held myself to an impossible standard when it comes to remaining objective.

Greg told me a bit about who he was, where he came from, and what he was looking for in the series he was starting. It was going to be a five- or six-race Midwest schedule, and he offered to pay more money than I was earning with the karting club, as well as covering any lodging costs. This sounded terrific to me.

There was just one catch: In addition to being his group's flagman, he also wanted me to be race director. As I've explained, this was not ideal for me; I had already shut down any thoughts of seeking the SLKA race-director job. But this was a regional series with better pay, travel expenses, and a chance to visit more tracks. My initial reaction was to say no, but instead I said yes to something I never would've looked for myself. My big concern was one I've already mentioned: that I'd have to speak at the driver's meeting.

In the weeks leading up to the season opener, I thought back to book reports I'd given in school. My second-grade teacher had to rescue me—as if she were a lifeguard and I were a swimmer swept out to sea—by reading my book report to the class. It was that dire, that traumatic for me. Why would I put myself through that? At the same time, I was beginning to learn that I was capable of things I'd never thought I could handle. Negative internal monologue be damned, I was going to do this, and do it right.

The CSSS and the Next Step

MY BURST OF CONFIDENCE DID NOT LAST. ANXIETY RETURNED and was raging out of control. Why did I sign up for this race-directing gig? Did I have the leadership qualities to even hold a drivers' meeting? And I still hadn't told Greg that I was on the autism spectrum. That was a big fear; in 2006, Asperger's wasn't a commonly known thing. How would Greg handle that discussion? How would I handle it? Why had I subjected myself to this guaranteed failure? Logically, it made no sense. I believed that there was no such thing as learning a skill set. A person either could do something, or they couldn't, and speaking was something I couldn't do. I knew that, and I was sure that Greg and all the racers would know that soon enough.

This new venture was called the Central States Super Series, and the season opener was at a place very familiar to me, West Quincy. I'd be making the 100-mile journey with Greg and Gary. Driving from our house to Greg's place that morning, I figured the ride north might give me time to help Greg lower his expectations of my skills. How's that for confidence? Yeah, this was going to be bad.

One good thing was that our timing was so well coordinated that there was no time for awkward pleasantries. Just as I opened my car doors at Greg's, he came out ready to go, and at the same time Gary pulled up. There was a quick flurry of activity moving bags from our vehicles to Greg's, and we were on the road headed to Quincy.

It was bound to happen, and it was the first thing we talked about: the black-flag situation that ended the '05 season. Gary mentioned it first, and wondered aloud if he should have been black-flagged for passing another kart under the yellow if he hadn't *seen* the yellow. But before long, he said that he'd only brought it up as a joke: "I was just messing with you, to see how you'd react." He added, "I always have enjoyed your work."

Whew!

What I thought might be a confrontational conversation was not confrontational at all. Gary said that other people who'd been at the track that day convinced him that he *had* passed under yellow, "so it was the right call."

Then Greg said, "Aaron, that's why I hired you. You made the call, backed it up, and didn't let it bother you." He was mistaken about it not bothering me, but that was okay.

This was the start of a new experience for me. Up to this point in my life, as you have read, almost everything I'd done had been a solo experience, with no real sense of being part of a team. For the first time, I was in a position where it wasn't only about how I did the job; there was also the social aspect, because you do have to have a certain level of cohesion if you're traveling and sharing time with coworkers for hours on end. The seeds planted on this first morning, on that ride with Greg and Gary, would grow into the branches that took me elsewhere.

We stopped for breakfast near Hannibal, Missouri. I smiled, because this trip reminded me of all the times my dad and I made the same drive when the St. Louis track was flooded. But as we continued on, a chill ran through me. My first driver's meeting was mere hours away.

It was about 7:30 a.m. when we pulled into the West Quincy track, officially called TNT Kartways. I couldn't help but feel at home—I'd been there so many times—and being on familiar ground did ease my nerves a bit. Intentionally or not, Greg had an idea that helped: He suggested that I walk the course as part of my race-director routine. I made a lap on foot, looking for anything that might be out of place. The track looked great, so I walked back to the pits. Soon enough, drivers, parents, and mechanics began to gather. Ready or not, it was showtime.

Greg spoke first, welcoming everyone to the opening round of the Central States Super Series. I stood to one side, holding pages of notes on things I wanted to address. By notes, I mean several pages covering every possible scenario and every possible outcome. When Greg handed things over to me, I was eager but not exactly polished.

Mind you, all of this is *my* perception of the first time conducting a drivers' meeting. I didn't know how it was for those listening, but I knew how uncomfortable I was. First, I had the most difficult time introducing myself. I was using a microphone, and each time I heard my voice I stumbled over my words. And once I finally did get rolling, I carried on too long. It might be a stretch to say that the snack bar went from serving breakfast items to the lunch menu while I was speaking, but I realized that I was citing far too many rules and procedures.

I was sure this meeting was a disaster that would forever tarnish my career. But when I finished, there was a round of applause. This confused me, but it sure helped my confidence.

The schedule had practice and qualifying on Saturday, with the races on Sunday. The first group on track was the kid-kart class, the smallest karts and least-powerful engines. The drivers range from ages 5 to 7, and the difference in skills can be immense, leading to some interesting moments on track. I once had a race leader mistakenly drive into the pits after taking the white flag. He had just one turn to go before the checkered flag but got overexcited and fooled himself into thinking he'd already won. That should have handed the win to the second-running driver, but he pitted, too … as did third place, and fourth, and so on. Only one kart remained on track, the slowest one in the field, but he was four laps down. For the first and only time in my life, I withdrew the white flag because the new leader still had four laps to run. Every time you think you've seen it all, you're reminded that you haven't.

Straight out of the pits, a kid somehow managed to "bicycle" onto two wheels and end up on his side. I threw the red flag, and a parent, who was a doctor, ran out to the kid who, naturally, was scared and screaming. The kid told the doctor that his neck hurt badly, so the doc told me to bring out the ambulance. Wait … ambulance?

Many tracks won't have an ambulance on-site for a practice day, and there wasn't one there on this day. I ran to Greg and said we needed an ambulance, so he went to the track owner, and somebody called 911. That's when the chaos started. Apparently, there was some kind of first responder spat between West Quincy, Missouri, and Quincy,

Illinois, where an ambulance was literally just two miles away. Instead, the dispatcher suggested that we call Palmyra, which is a 20-minute drive by car. So that call was made, and we waited, and waited, and waited.

An hour went by, and the kid was still lying on his back where his kart had come to rest, with the doctor keeping his head and neck stable. Aside from the pain of the crash, the kid had to be incredibly uncomfortable lying in a strange position with all of his equipment on.

Back and forth I went, from the kid to the track to help Greg. Each time I went past a group of people, I'd be bombarded with questions. There was a grave concern as to why there wasn't an ambulance already on-site, and questions about whether we should continue this practice day. For a rookie race director, this was not a great day.

After 90 minutes, the track redialed 911, and we were once again told that the Quincy ambulance wouldn't cross the river.

Shortly after that, an ambulance did arrive—from where, I'm still not sure—and the injured boy was finally whisked off to get the proper care. Thankfully, he had no injuries other than some bumps and bruises, and he was back at the track the next day. We did resume practice, after assurances that if we needed another ambulance, one would be dispatched without delay.

Sunday's program went off without any major issues. One parent asked why I hadn't issued a penalty to a driver he believed had bumped his child's kart off the track. I explained what I saw, and the parent ranted a bit about the other kid. I listened intently, nodded my head, and was sympathetic to how he felt.

Somehow this felt ... *natural*.

I assured this father that I'd keep an eye on the driver in question but added that if the same incident occurred again in the same way, I'd stick to my belief that the incident was "just racing." Later, the man thanked me for listening, and said that he respected that I wouldn't change the way I called something just because a parent was complaining.

On the ride home, Greg said that he'd heard nothing but praise for the way Sunday had gone. I'd passed my race-director's rookie test. The season was off to a great start.

Finding Kansas ... City

IN THE WEEK AFTER THE CSSS SEASON OPENER, MY DUTIES expanded. We decided that I would generate race reports and previews for the series, and I liked the idea that this would put to good use my newfound love of writing. There wasn't much of a break before the next event in Carrollton, Missouri. Probably because Carrollton is in the western part of the state, and not exactly a booming metropolis known to all, our schedule read that it was in Kansas City.

It was an exciting time for me, because my dad had sent a compilation of my writings to a researcher in New York City. He said that she had been shocked with how candid I'd been in some of the revelations that I put forth, and that kept me motivated to continue my writing journey. Oddly, after this weekend, my two writing interests—racing and my autism—would collide.

Only a week after I'd been so nervous about the trip to West Quincy with Greg and Gary, I looked forward to traveling with them to Carrollton. Riding west on I-70, I opened up about being on the autism spectrum. That led to some predictable "like Rain Man" questions; for most people, autism was still shrouded in mystery. But as we rolled across the Missouri countryside, I gained confidence in explaining my strengths, challenges, and joys.

Saturday's practice and qualifying went by without issue, and, happily, so did my Sunday drivers' meeting. During the morning warmups, two drivers chatted with me between their sessions. We talked karting, Formula 1, IndyCar; it was a nice, lively conversation that I enjoyed.

The racing went well, aside from an incident here and there. But remember what I said about how people will blame race directors for everything, even the weather? On this day, there was a visible shower off to the west; it was just hanging around, with no clear direction. After each feature race, we held podium ceremonies right away, but we stuck to our schedule. Well, one parent was irate with me for not hurrying things more; I was blamed in advance for "the carnage to come." I'll never forget the disdain on this man's face as he berated me. It never did rain, but I realized that a race director can be blamed even for weather that *doesn't* happen.

At the end of the program, the two drivers I'd talked with earlier approached me again. What happened next was interesting, but also sad. Now that I was off-duty—having finished my day's work as flagman and race director—I was a different person from the one they'd talked with earlier. All I seemed able to say to them was "yes" and "no" and, at the most, "I don't know." It was proof that as long as I was playing a role, in this case a race official, I was able to converse with an ease that normally isn't there. Now I was just me again.

On the inside, I was crying. I wanted to be the same person they'd talked with just a few hours earlier, but my body and brain wouldn't allow it. My heart broke when one of them asked, "Are you sure you're the same person I was talking to earlier?"

I'm sure everyone behaves slightly differently in different situations, but to go from a sense of complete freedom in conversation to a feeling of being chained and unable to respond, well, that's drastic. I wish I could have answered his question in a way he understood, by saying something like, "Yes, I'm the same person, but it's a more hectic and open-ended environment right now, and this isn't easy for me."

On the ride back to St. Louis, Greg and Gary tried to converse with me, but all I could think about was those two drivers trying to figure out what had happened to me. As we got to Kingdom City, a tire blew on Greg's trailer, and we spent hours at a truck stop trying to get it fixed. Sitting there, I realized that I couldn't wait to write something. Everyone was asleep when I finally got home, so I sat down at the computer and started writing about how Carrollton, during the racing program, had been a place where I felt normal, and everything made sense.

But as I wrote, I realized that "Carrollton" didn't have the right ring to it. I looked up at the ceiling, then to my race director's notepad on a tray to my right. At the top, it said, "Round 2: Kansas City." I started changing all the mentions of Carrollton to "Kansas City." Again, it just wasn't right. I dropped the "City," and ended up with just "Kansas." I didn't know it yet, but I was well into writing my first book … and now you know where the title came from.

I never did see those two drivers again. I wonder if they're aware of the role they played in my mission to reach people with my words and speeches on this topic.

—————— Hope, Desire, and Pain ——————

MY DAD AND I WOULD BE ATTENDING OUR 10TH STRAIGHT Indy 500 in 2006. But a couple of days before we headed to Indianapolis, my dad took me to go see Temple Grandin speak in St. Louis. If you don't know of Dr. Grandin, she is easily the most famous autism authority and has published numerous books and articles on the subject. She is also a Doctor of Animal Sciences who, among many other things, revolutionized the way cattle chutes operated by using her visual thinking to simulate it from the cow's perspective. She has earned honorary degrees from universities all over the world and has even been on *Time* magazine's list of the 100 Most Influential People in the world. Without a doubt, she was the first autistic person I knew of who had ever been successful.

My dad had tried and tried to get me to read her books, or any of those written by Dr. Tony Attwood, a British psychologist whose specific focus has been Asperger's syndrome. But that website I'd looked at on the night of my diagnosis continued to be my only source of information. Why take time out of my day to study and read about this condition when failure was a guarantee? But having me attend the Temple Grandin speech was a smart move by my dad, because sitting there made me a captive audience; you can't close a speech and put it down, or ignore it altogether, the way you can do with a book.

As she spoke about overcoming her challenges, I thought that maybe someday my words would be published; maybe I'd be on a stage somewhere explaining my life and insights; maybe I could give people hope. It's odd I thought about hope because, all too often, I would only use that word when dealing with a sense of hopelessness.

A few days later we went to Indianapolis for the 500, and for the first time I became an emotional mess during pre-race ceremonies. For those that have been to the 500, or even watched it on television, that pre-race time is almost akin to a religious service. During "Back Home Again in Indiana" I thought about everyone in those grandstands, in the infield, and in the pits who had attended the 500 with their dads, like I had done and continued to do. It got to me, and briefly I found myself crying. There's no getting around it: Indy is so much more than a race; for those who love it, it's ingrained in who they are.

As quickly as they came, the tears were brushed away. The command to start engines and the slow buildup of the pace laps always replace sentimentality with tension. Finally, there's the release when the 33 cars, in 11 rows of three, take the green flag.

And the 2006 Indianapolis 500 was an amazing race. We were seated in turn three, a great spot to watch the breathtaking duel between Sam Hornish Jr. and Marco Andretti. With less than two laps to go, right in front of us, Hornish attempted an inside pass for the lead, but Marco shut the door. Hornish's left-side tires just clipped the infield grass, and for an instant I was sure they would both careen into the outside wall. Hornish lost ground but was undeterred; he chased down Marco on the final lap, and won the sprint from turn four to the checkered flag.

It was an incredible day, and I couldn't stop thinking about how badly I wanted to be a part of that race someday. I clung to a thin thread of hope that I'd be behind the wheel, racing at 230 miles per hour someday, but one way or another, I knew I wanted a life in racing.

Coincidentally, when I got home, I saw an ad for a new indoor karting track in St. Louis. Maybe it could provide the job I was looking for. In an uncharacteristic act, I cold-called the place and set up an interview. I met with the owner, who reviewed my application and said he was impressed with my 11 years working at a track.

The man said, "Aaron, you're the most qualified applicant I've seen. With your knowledge and experience, I should be working for *you*."

I felt like I had nailed this interview, and, as I'm sure you've sensed by now, I don't often experience that sense of sheer confidence.

And then, in an instant, that confidence dissolved into

self-loathing when he wrapped up with these words: "I can offer you a corner position for minimum wage."

Minimum wage. I tried not to show emotion. Slowly, methodically, I stood up and left.

Having believed for so long that failure is a guarantee, it had been a thrill to hear such positivity about my qualifications, my knowledge, my experience. I knew I should have a great job, not because I was entitled it but because I'm sharp and I'm dedicated. But hearing that I was only worth *minimum* wage was like five tons of bricks being dumped onto my shoulders.

When I got outside and into my car, I called my dad. Whatever words I managed to say turned into screams of agony, and I pounded my fist on the steering wheel.

That day, the future became something I truly feared. Outside of race-directing a regional kart series and a local karting club, what could I do? Everything seemed impossible. I wondered if it would be easier to just accept what I thought was my fate, give up racing, and live in my dad's basement for the rest of time.

No, the story didn't end there. You already know that. But I can't sugarcoat the feeling I had; it sucked, and that's as eloquent as I can be about it.

An Old Flagman, Photos, a New Job, and a Christmas Party

IT TOOK A MONTH, BUT THE INDOOR-KARTING INTERVIEW slid into the near-past, instead of feeling ever-present. It helped that I had a Central States Super Series race in

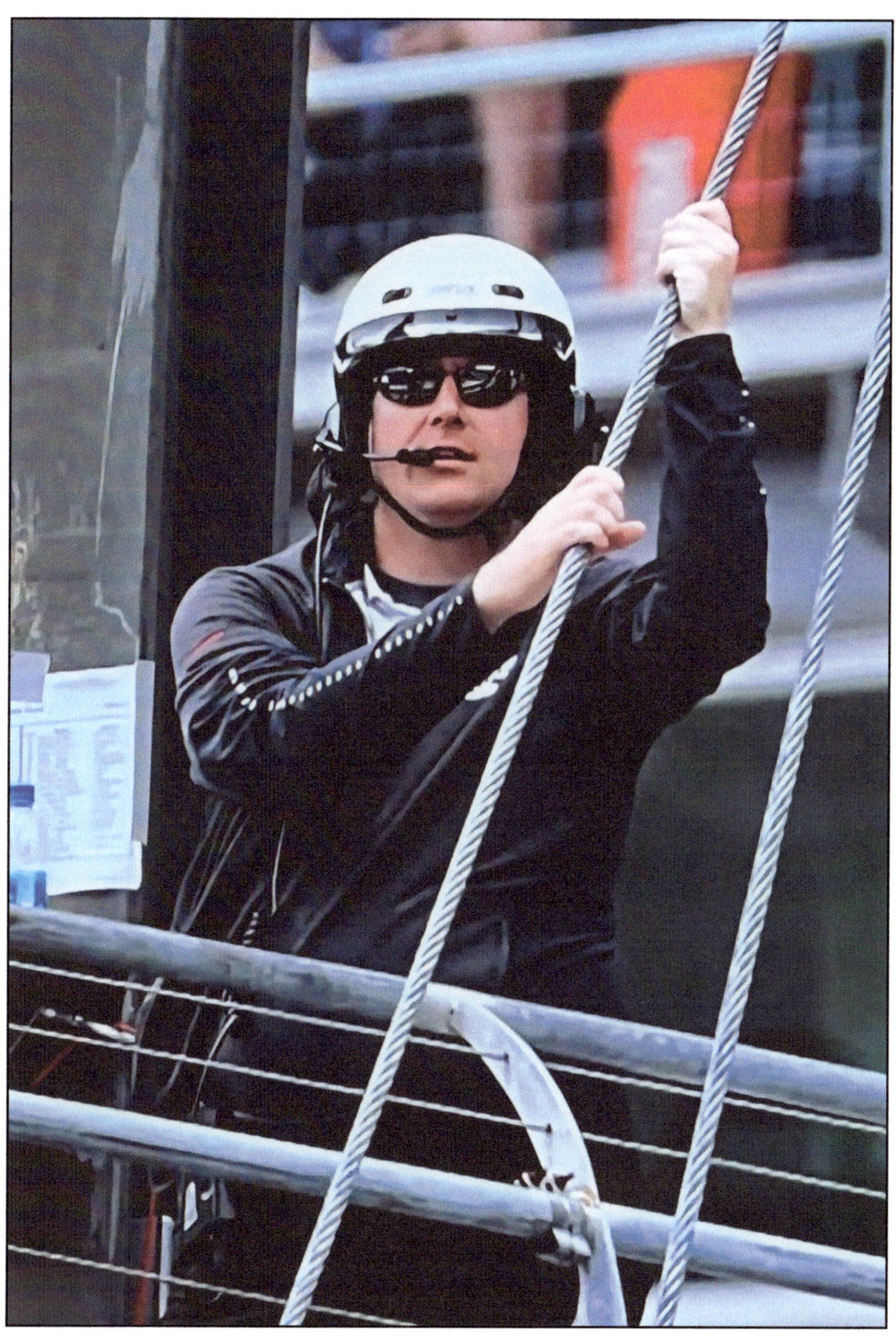

Aaron in the Indianapolis Motor Speedway flagstand.

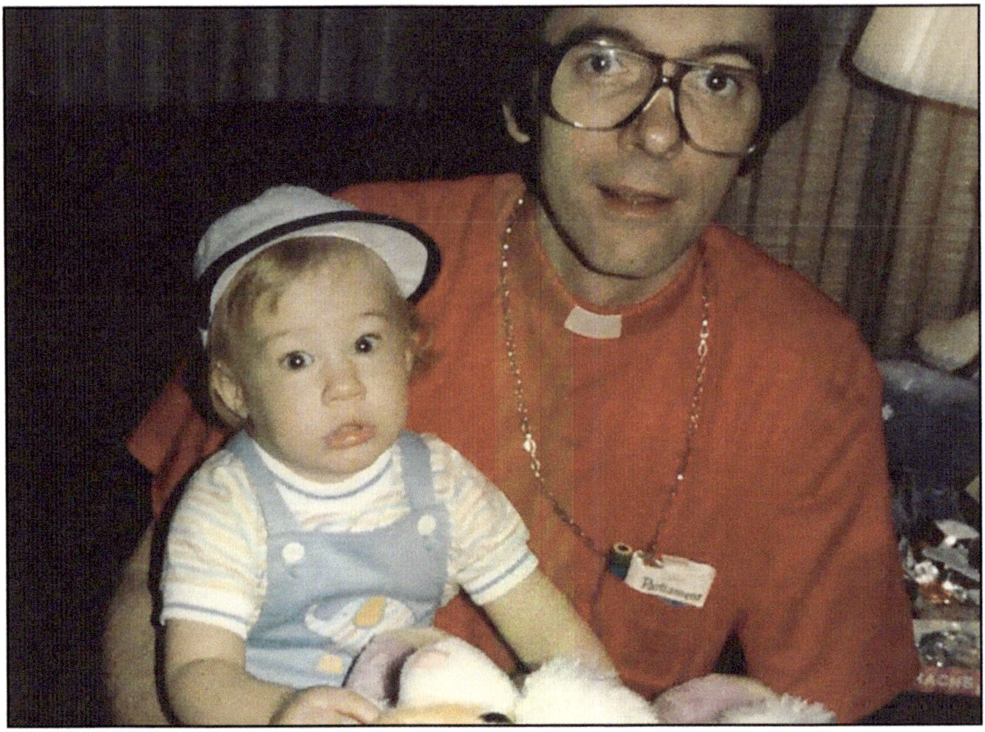

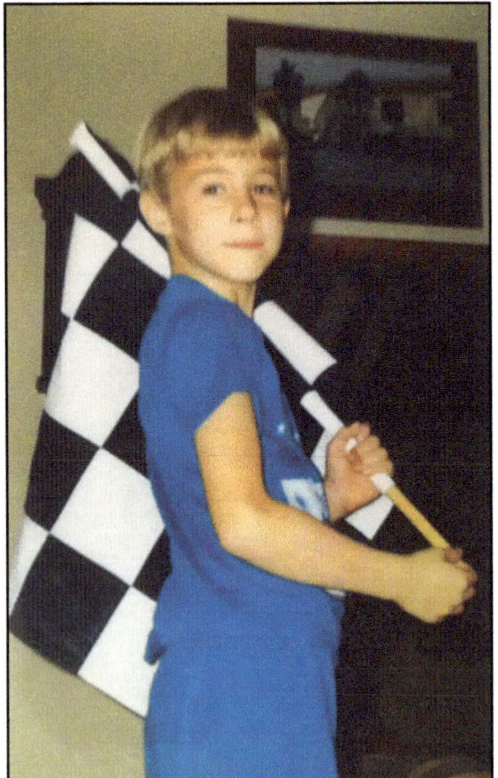

Above: Dad Jim Likens with 10-month-old Aaron.

Left and Below: Destiny in the making. Aaron on the day he received his checkered flag from longtime Indy 500 starter Duane Sweeney.

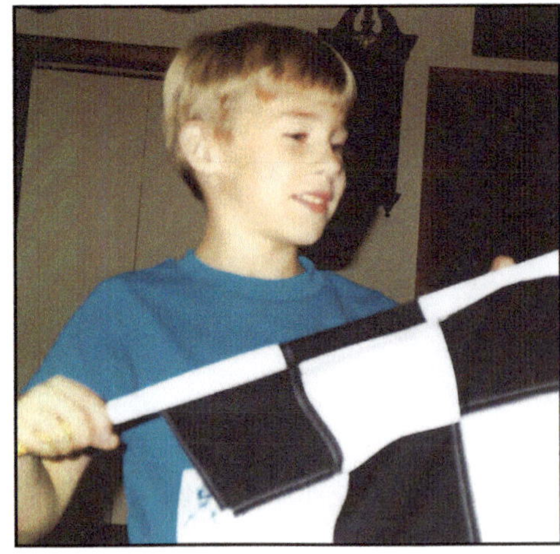

Aaron's racing roots at St. Louis County, Widman Park, the karting track near St. Louis.

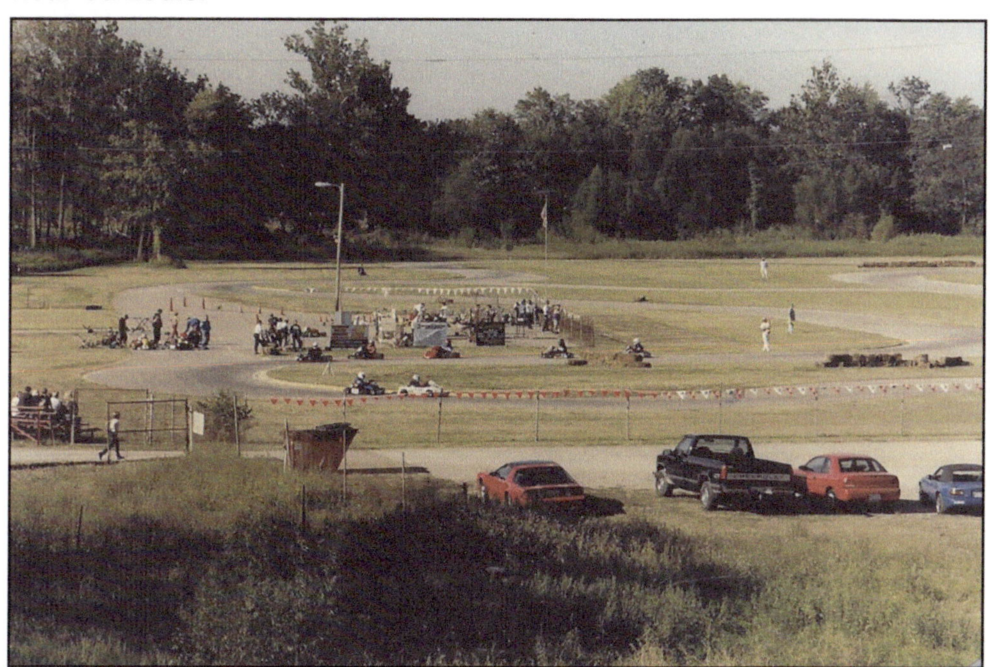

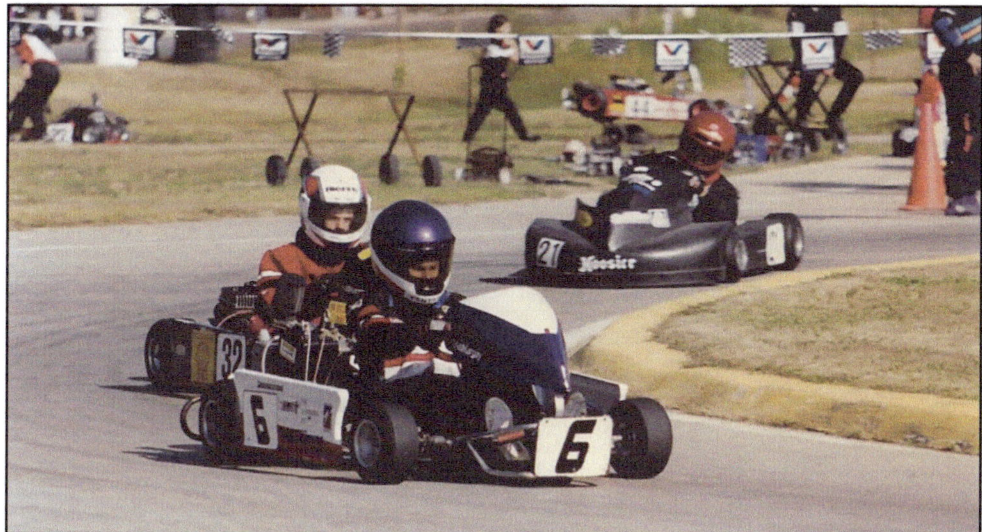

Aaron holds the lead in the hairpin at Widman.

Flagging at the Widman track.

Aaron with Frankie Neidenbach
at a St. Louis Karting Association
race, 1997.

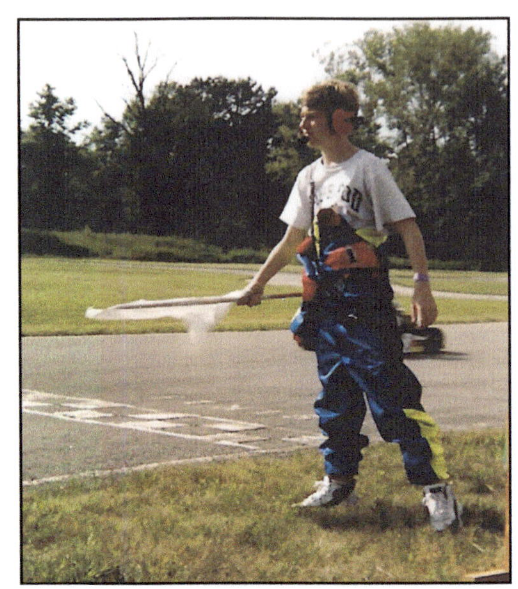

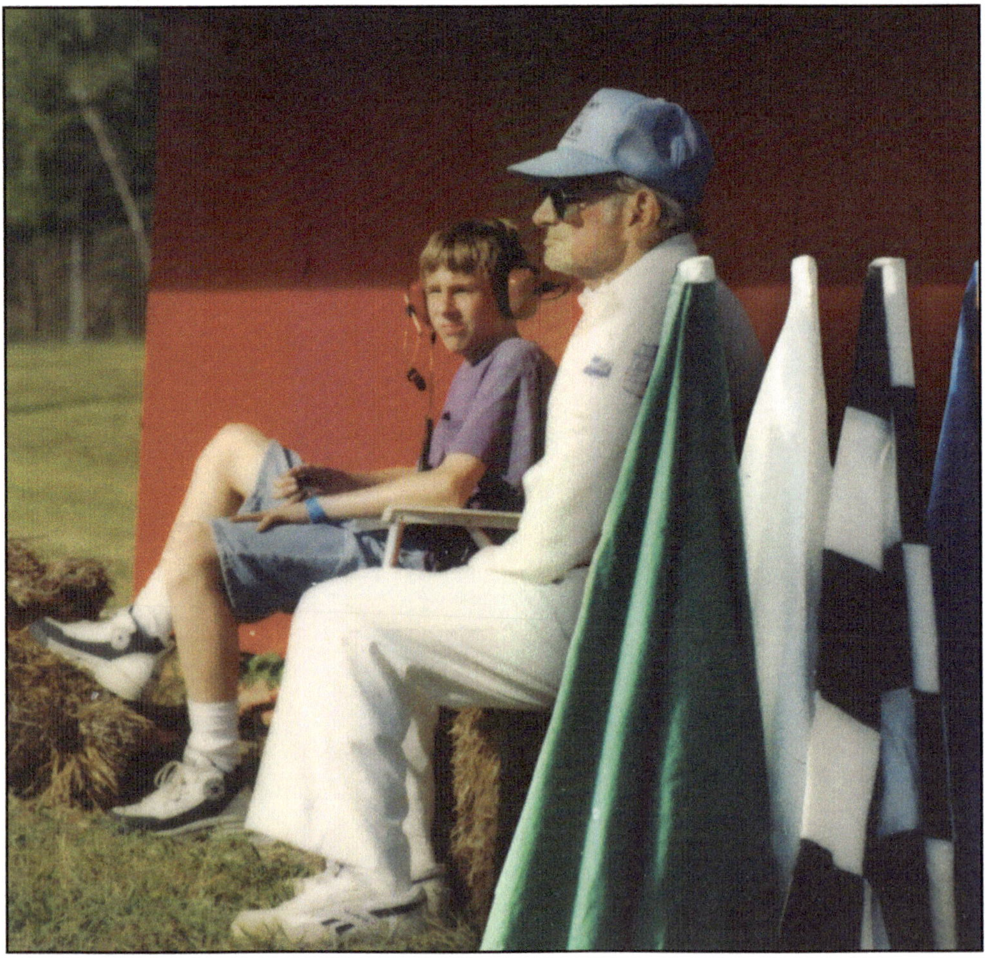

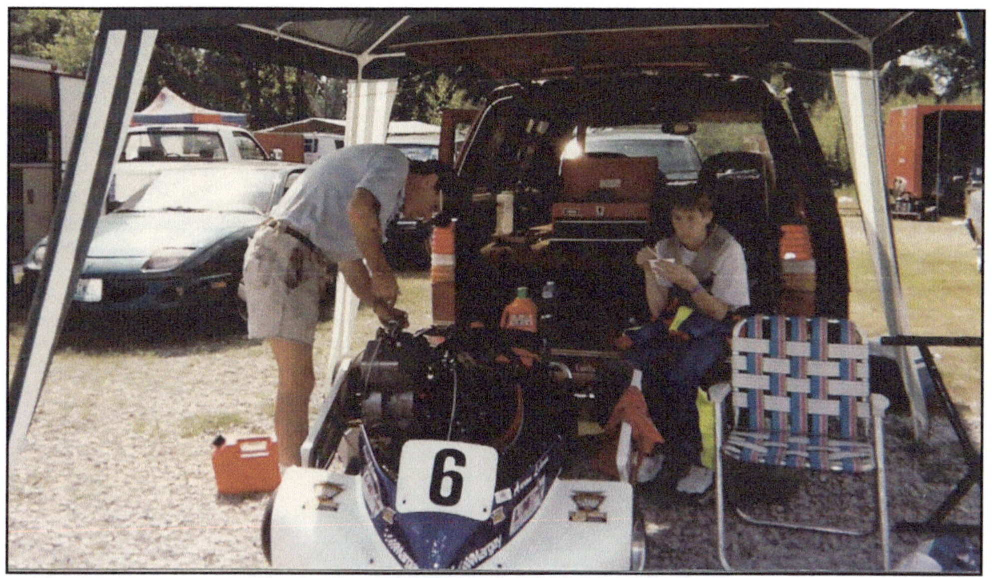

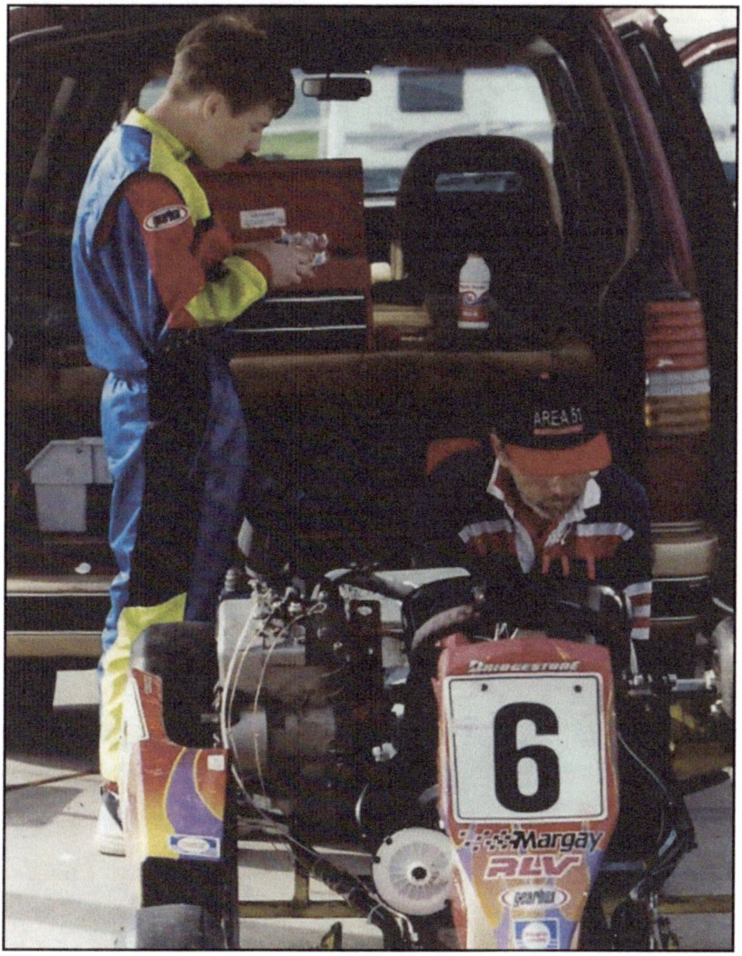

Lunch in the pits at Widman and West Quincy.

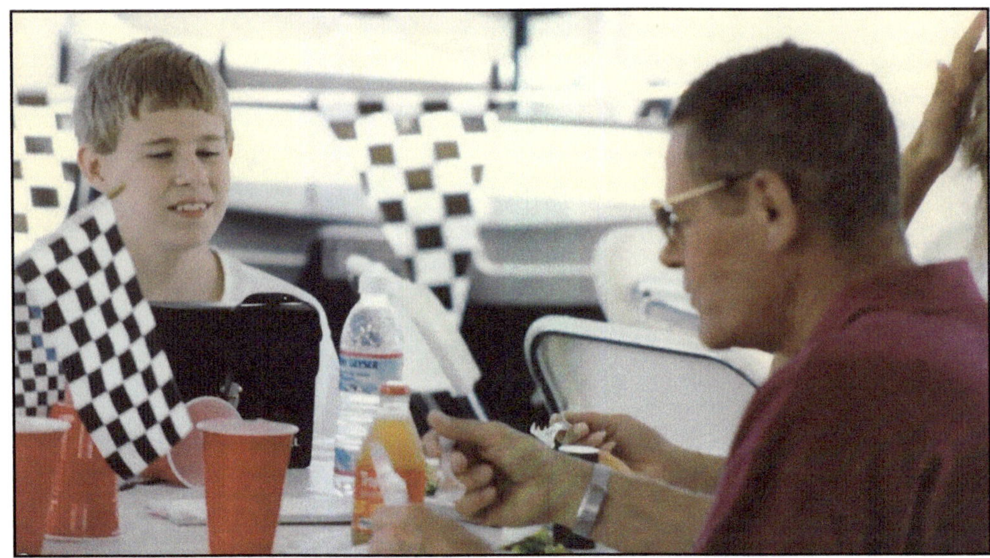

Above: Breakfast with a legend. Aaron and three-time Indy 500 winner Bobby Unser share a table at Las Vegas Motor Speedway in 1996.

Below: Jonathan Byrd's VisionAire car on the grid at Las Vegas Motor Speedway, 1996.

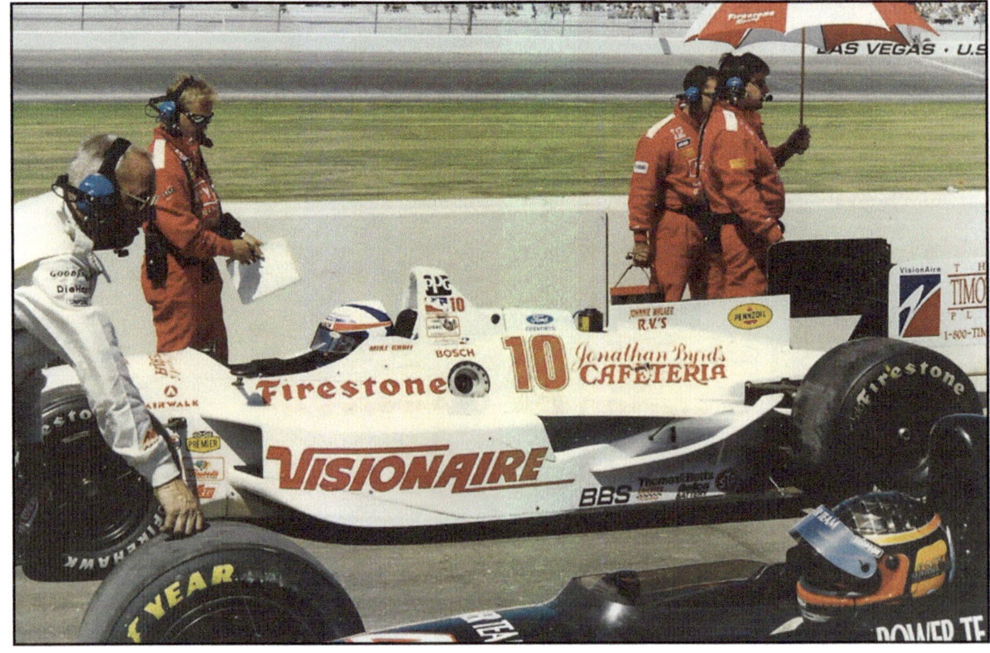

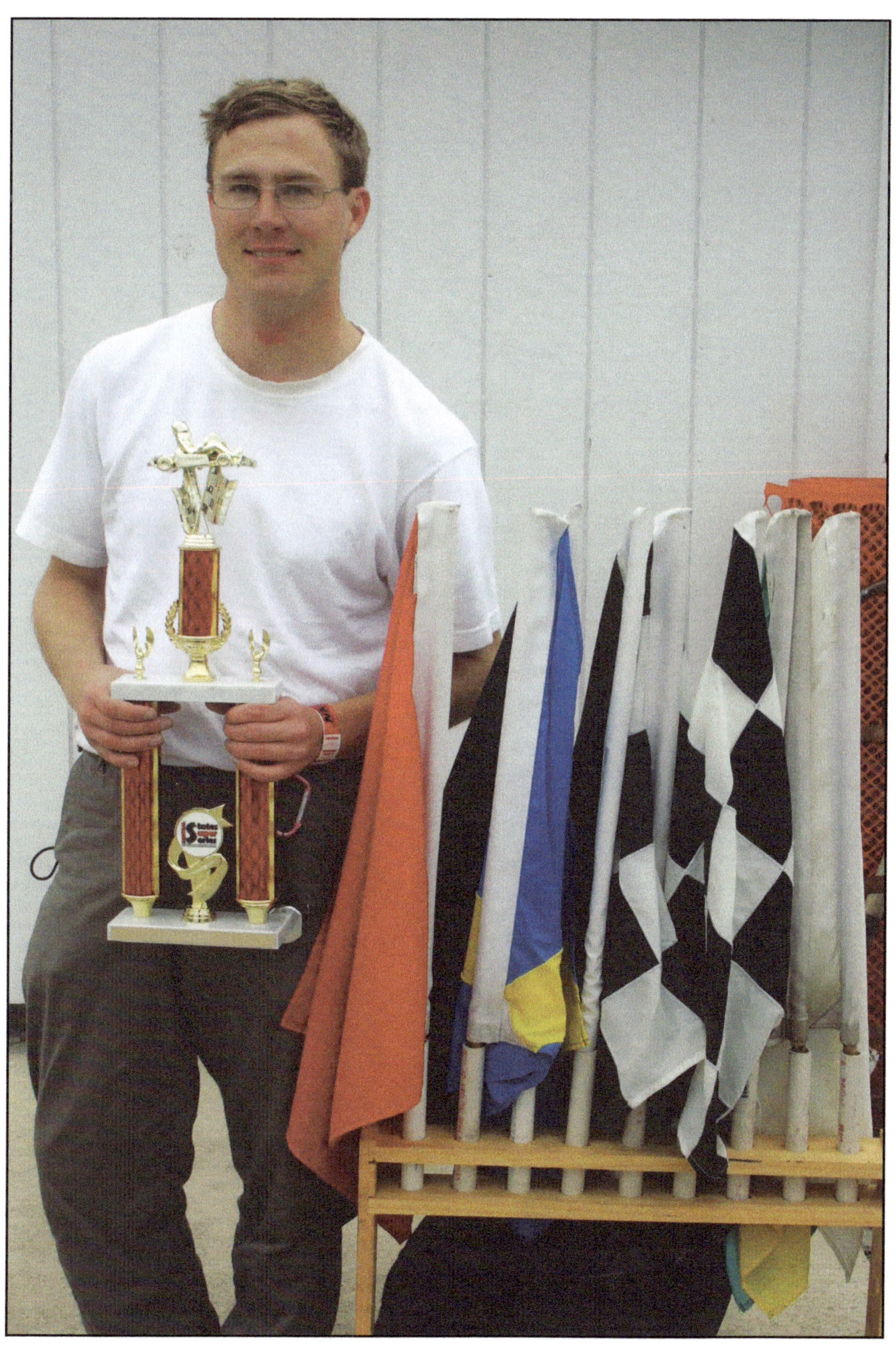

Double duty, picking up karting trophies and flagging races, too.

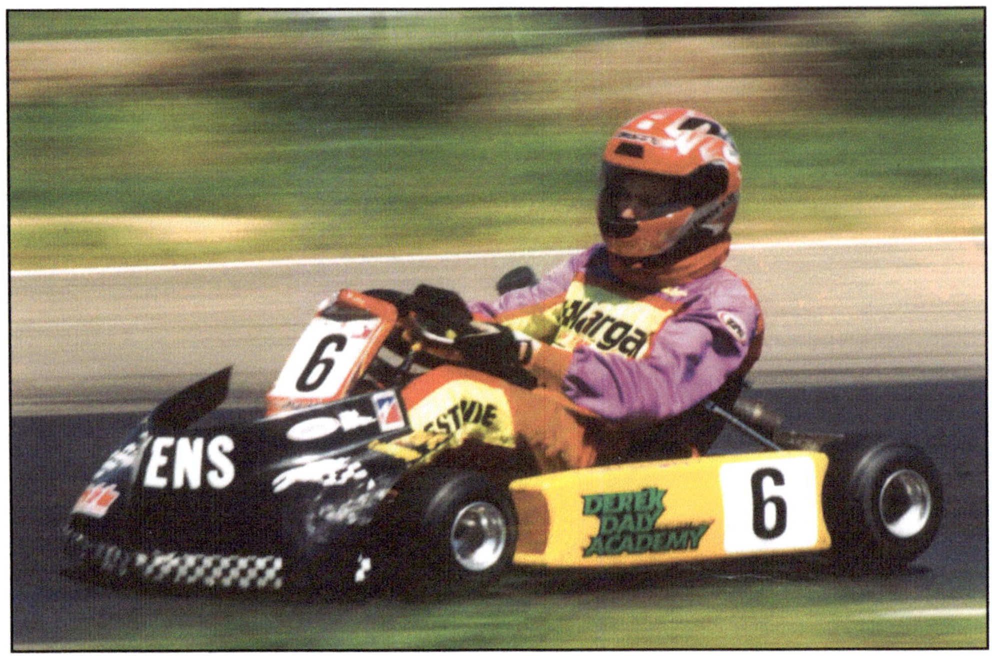

Above: Aaron on his way to victory at the Mid-State Kart Club track, Springfield, Illinois.

Below: Climbing the ladder as a racer, Aaron had stints as both a student and an instructor at the Derek Daly Academy.

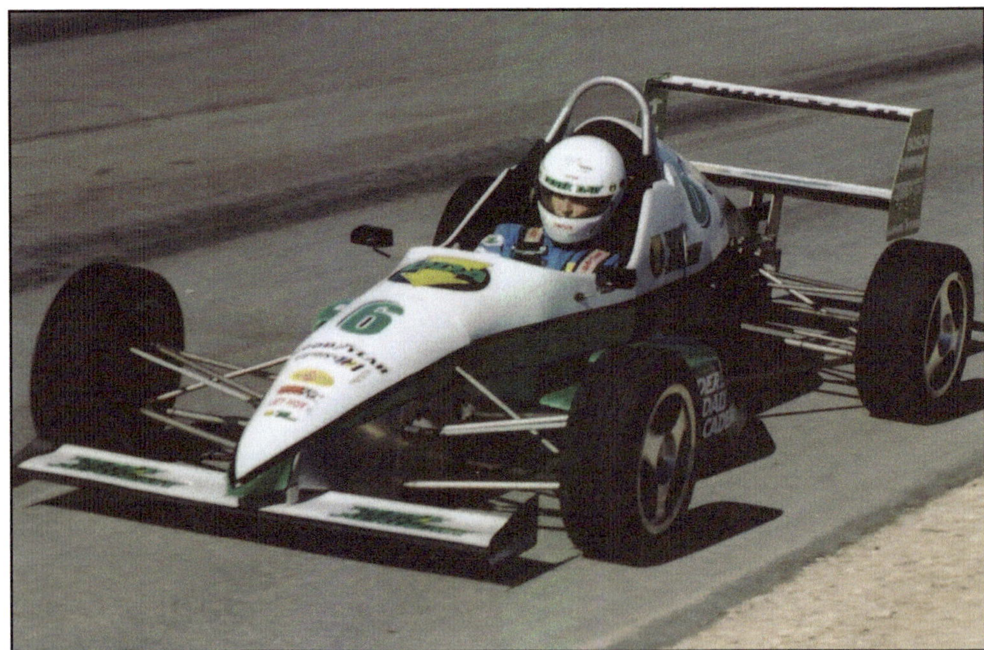

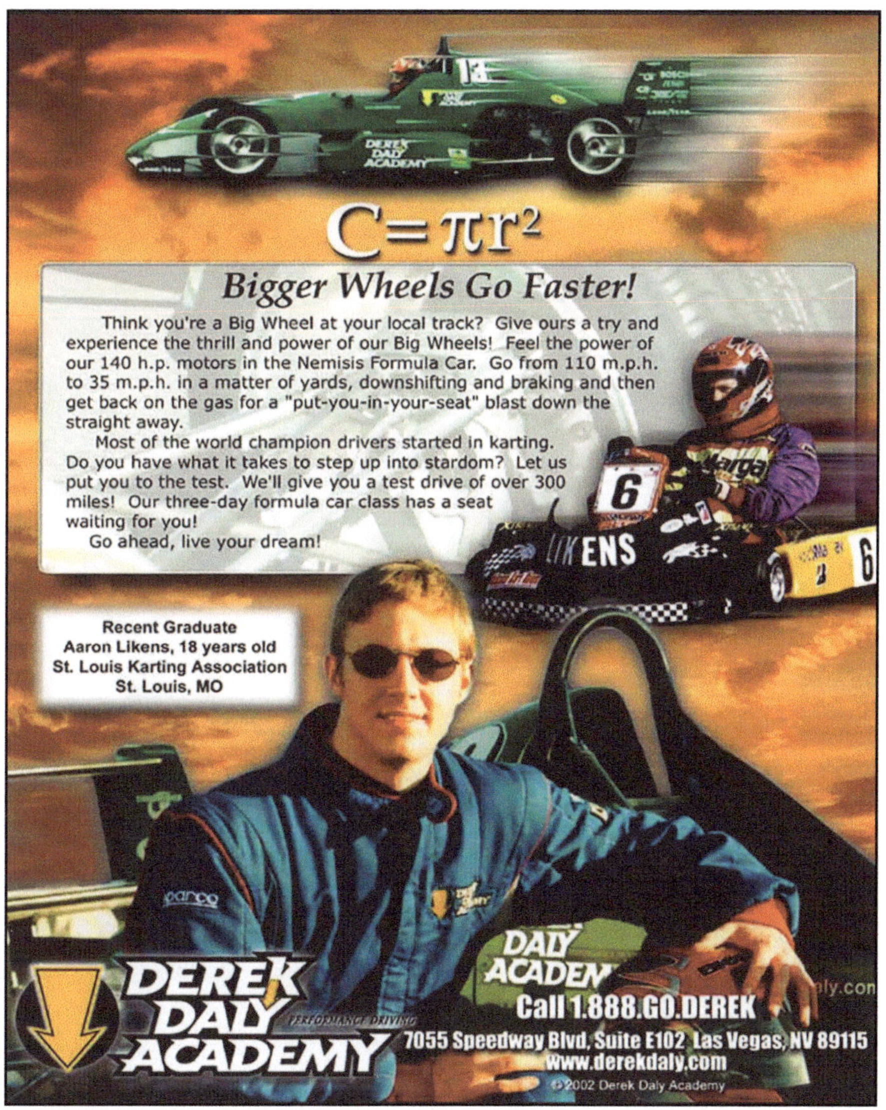

Aaron was featured in an advertisement for the Derek Daly Academy.

Aaron flagging his first SKUSA SuperNationals in 2008.

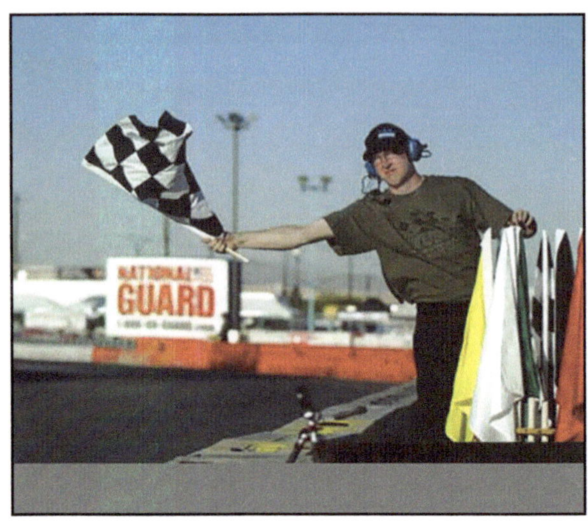

SKUSA boss Tom Kutscher shares a moment with Aaron at the SuperNats, the Super Bowl of karting.

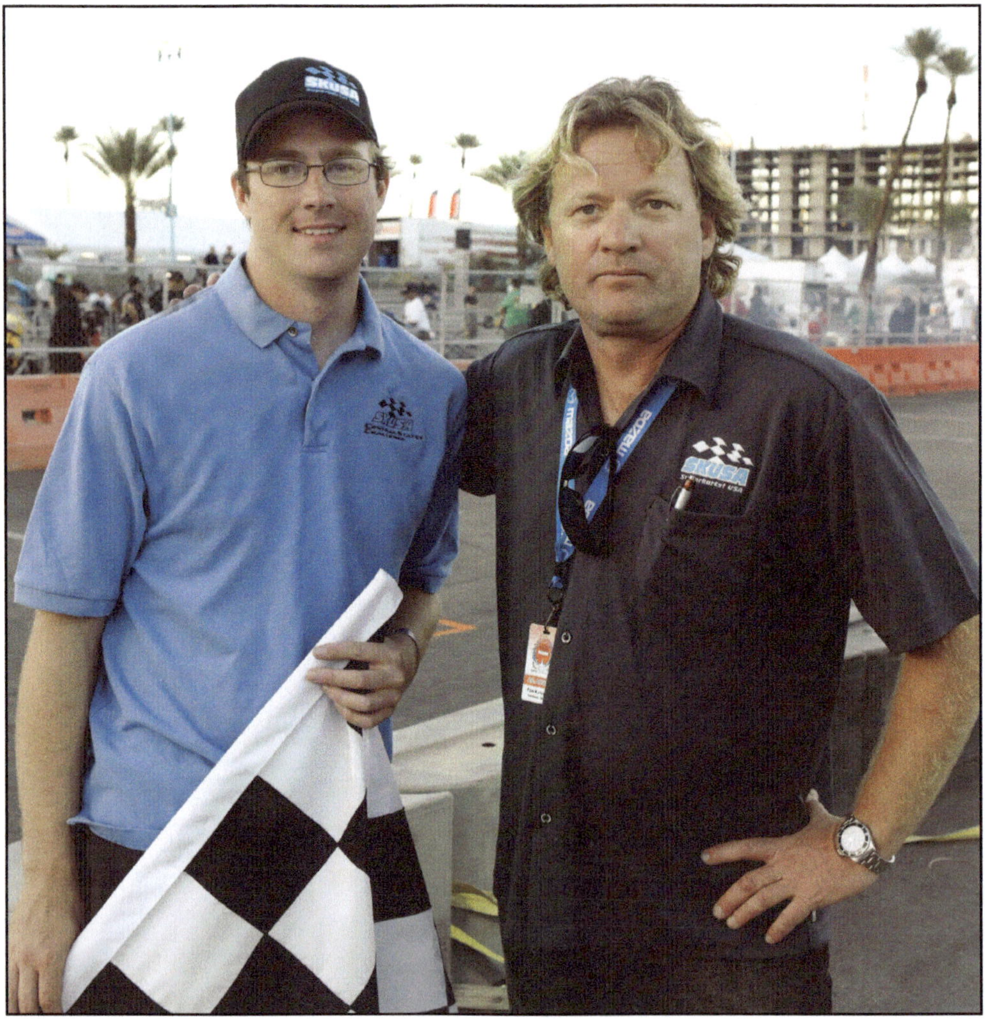

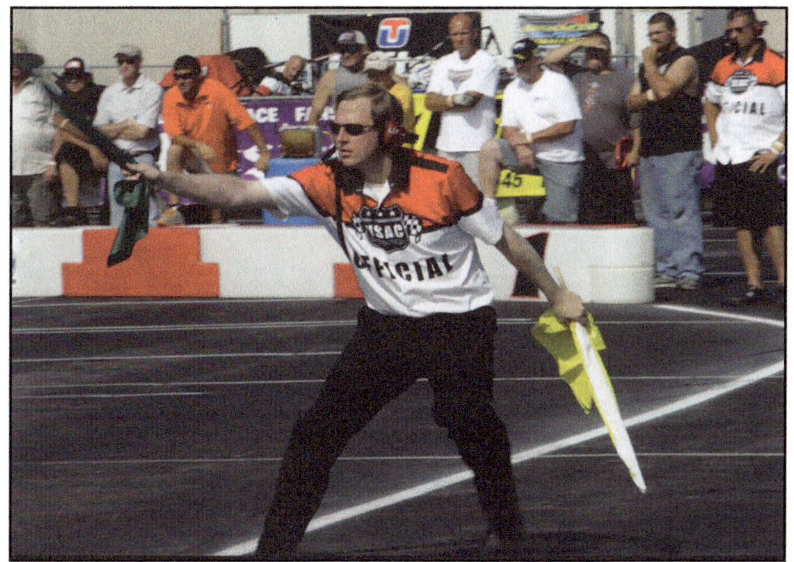

Above: Aaron's first USAC .25 Midgets race, the 2010 Battle at the Brickyard. *(Craig Somers Photo)*

Below: Aaron (left) and Kyle McCain formed a tight bond in their days on the USAC .25 Midget trail.

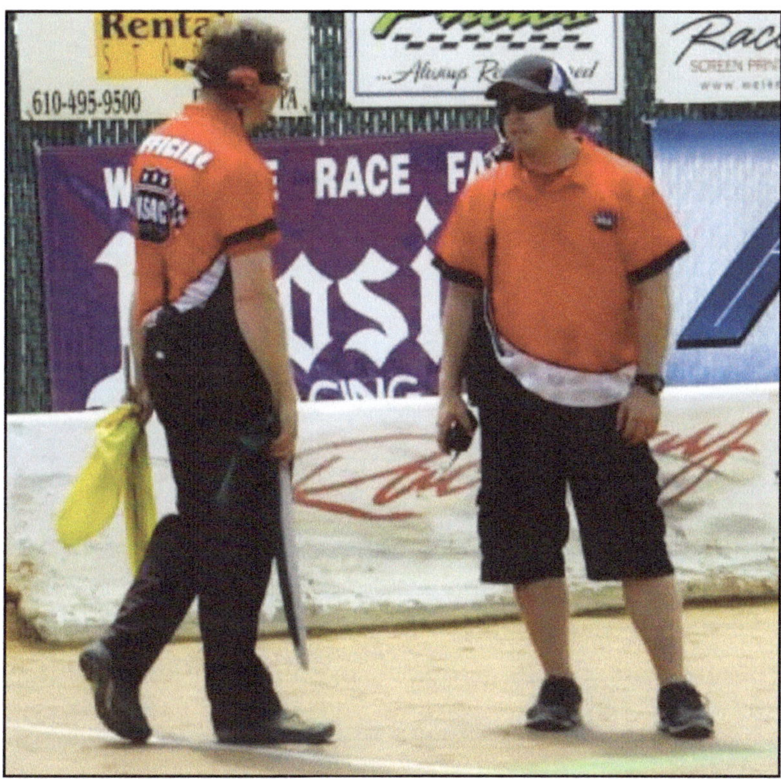

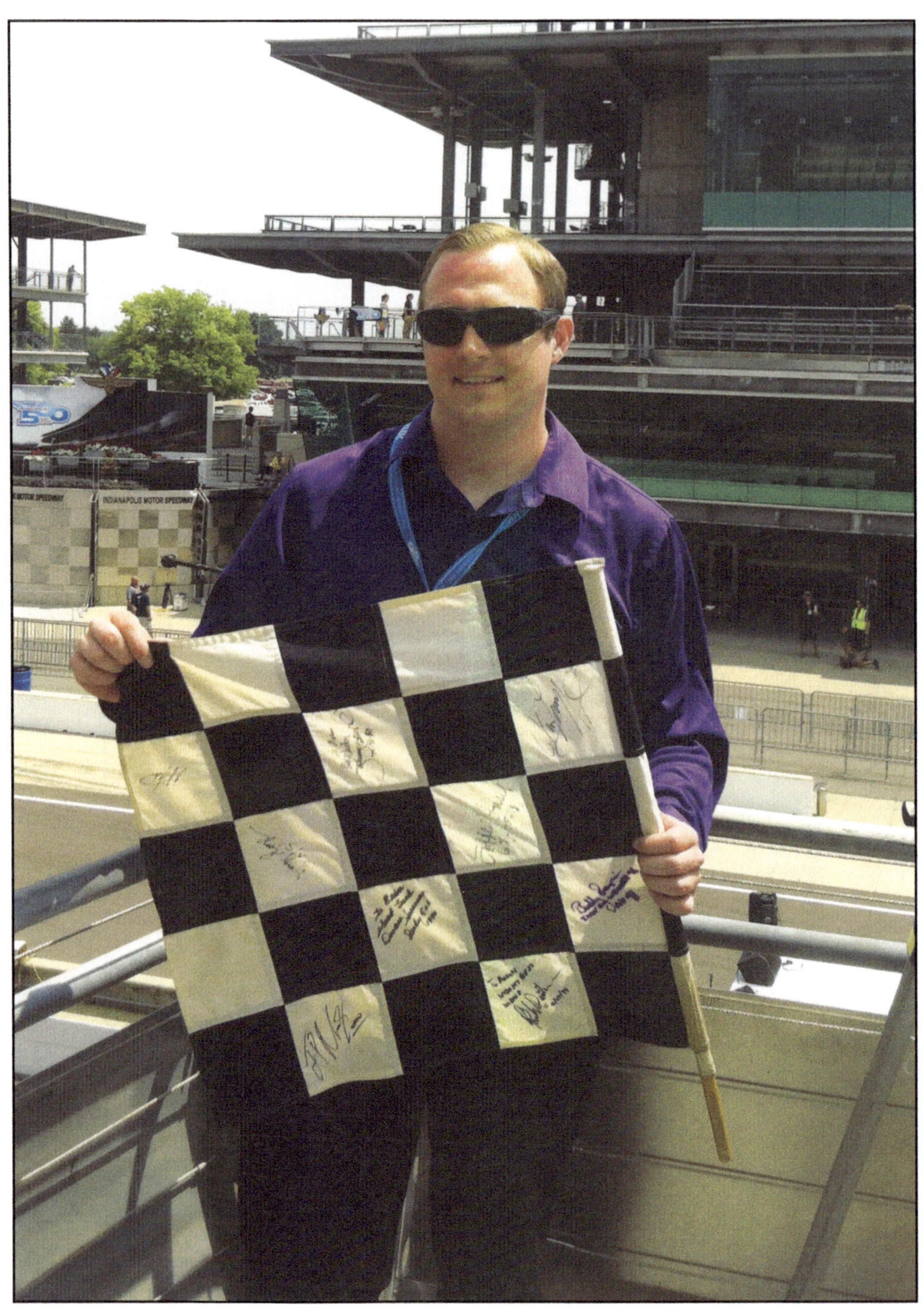

In 2012, as part of a series of video blogs highlighting autism awareness, Aaron visited the IMS flagstand with the flag he'd been given by
Duane Sweeney.

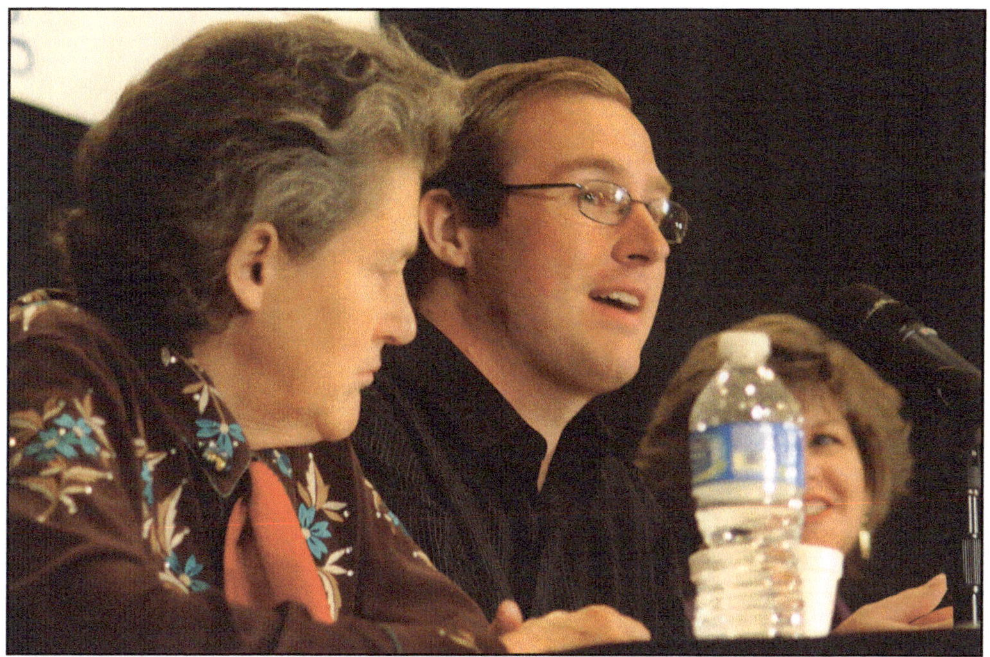

Above: Aaron in 2011, as part of a panel discussion with Dr. Temple Grandin, famed autism-advocacy pioneer.

Lower left: Aaron with Ron Ekstrand at a St. Louis Cardinals game when Aaron threw out the first pitch.

Lower right: In 2012 Aaron was honored with the Missouri Champions of Mental Health Award.

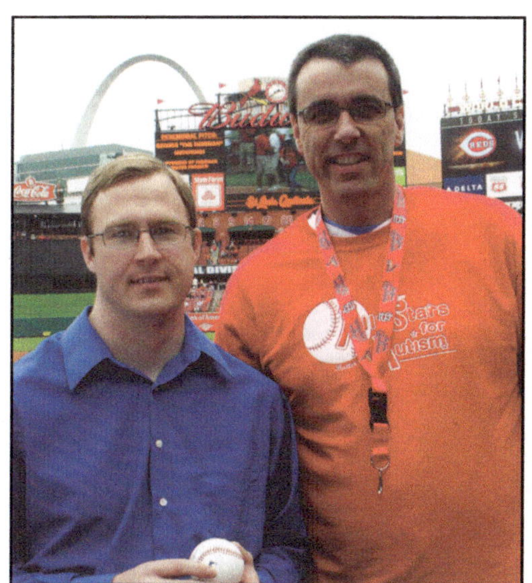

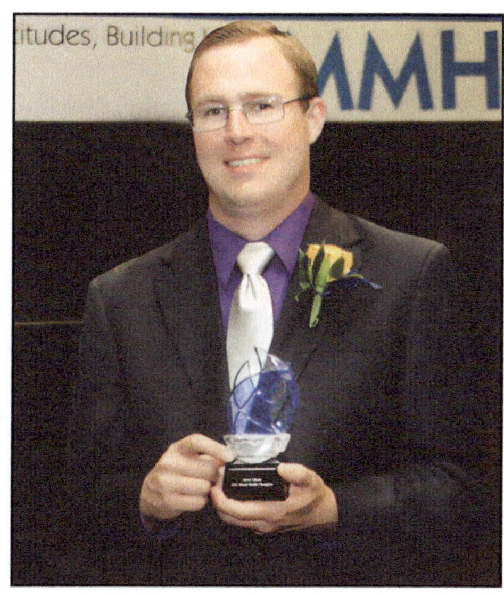

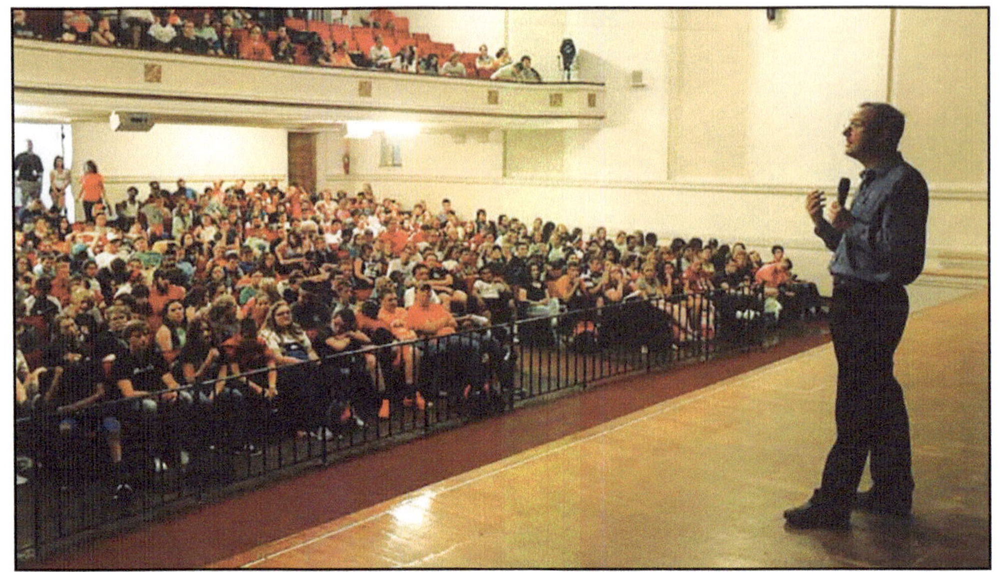

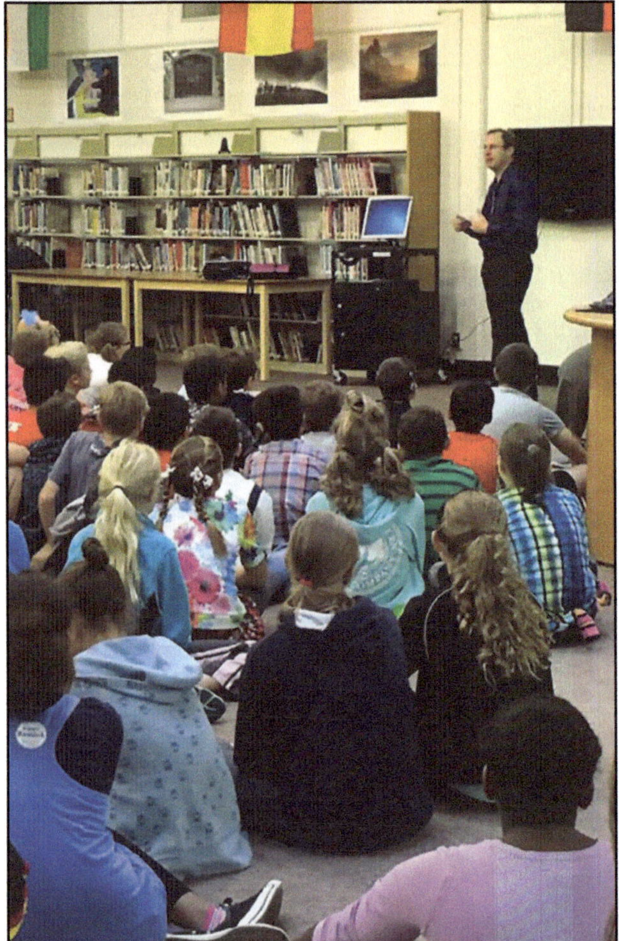

Above: Passing it along. Aaron makes a point during a presentation at Hannibal High School, Hannibal, Missouri.

Left: Aaron also spoke to younger children about autism, here a third-grade class.

Opposite page above: Aaron's inspiring story has led to numerous media interviews, including this one with KSDK-TV in St. Louis.

Opposite page below: Back where it all began. This neighborhood rock was Aaron's first "flagstand." A local TV interview included a trip to the rock.

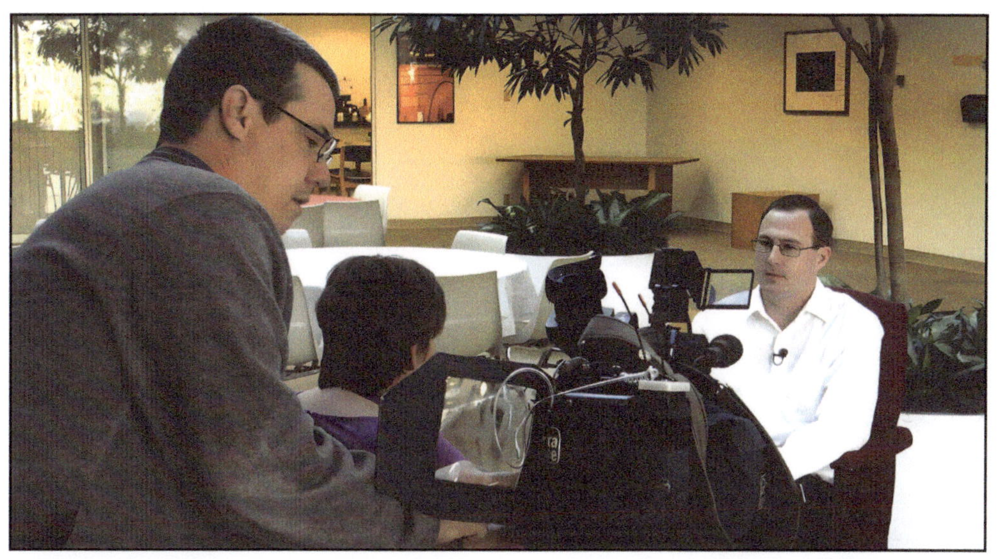

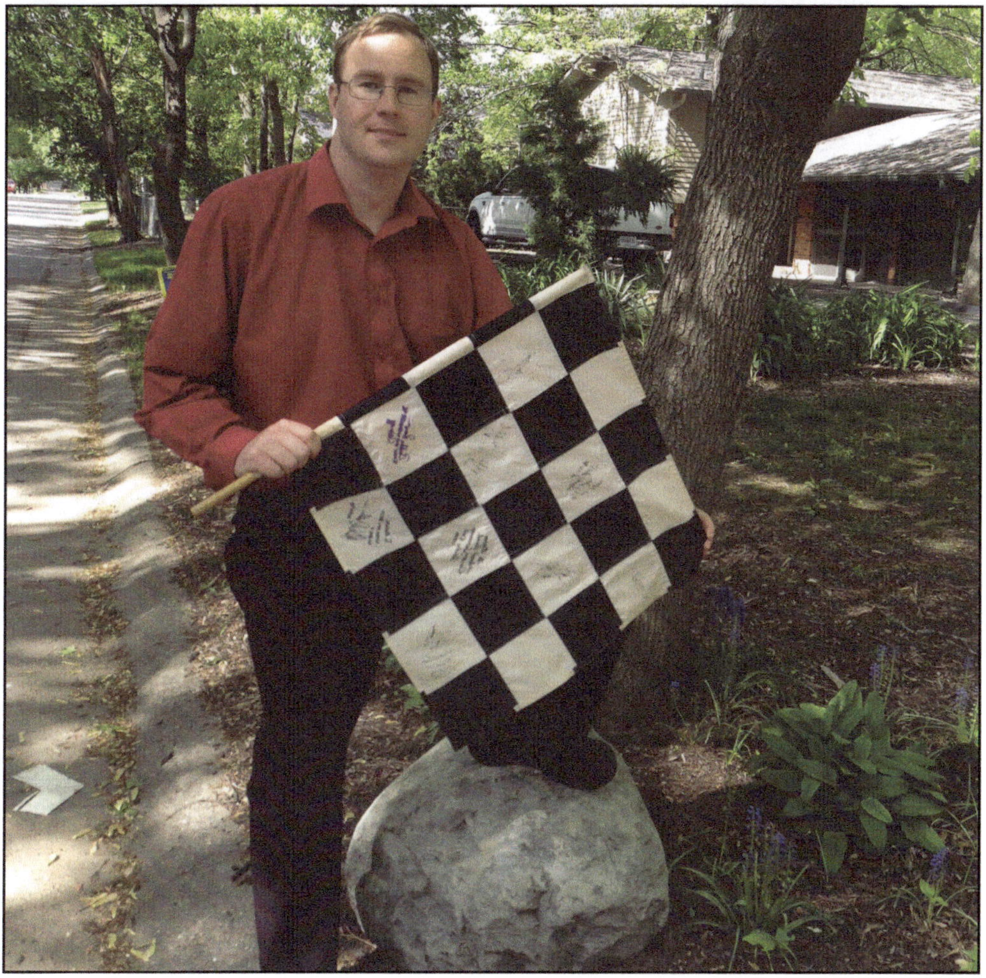

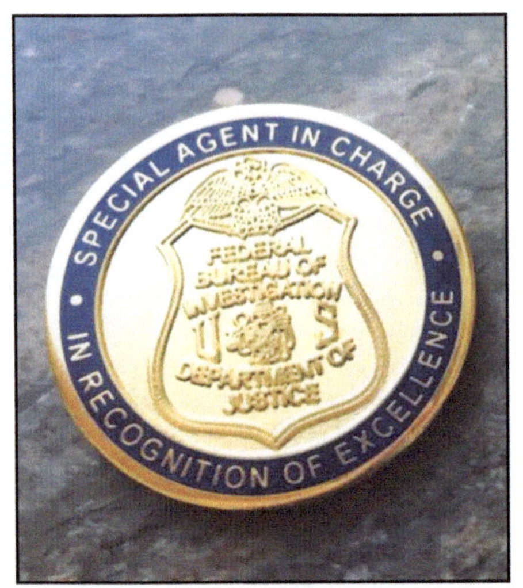

Aaron was a popular speaker with the FBI and as thanks for one of his presentations to FBI agents, Aaron was given this "Recognition of Excellence" challenge coin.

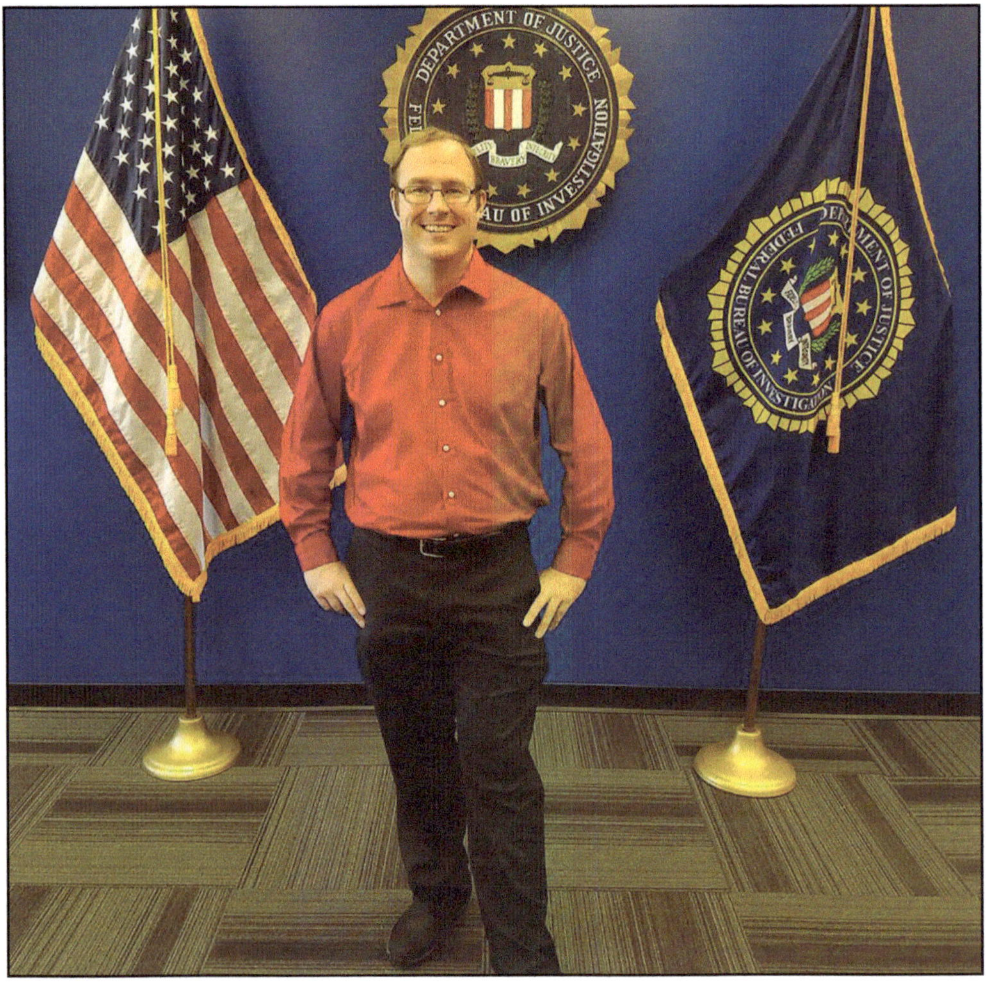

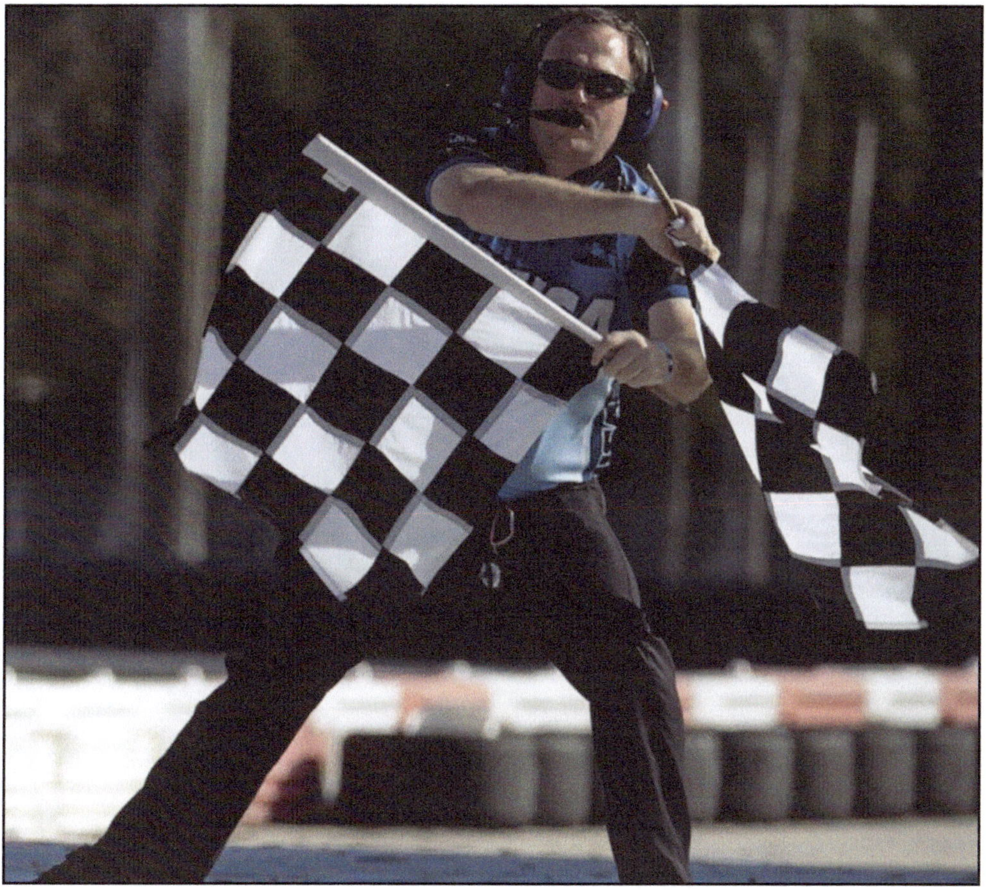

Above: A SKUSA double checker. *(On-Track Productions Photo)*

Below: Night racing at the SuperNationals, Las Vegas. *(Matt Fink Photo)*

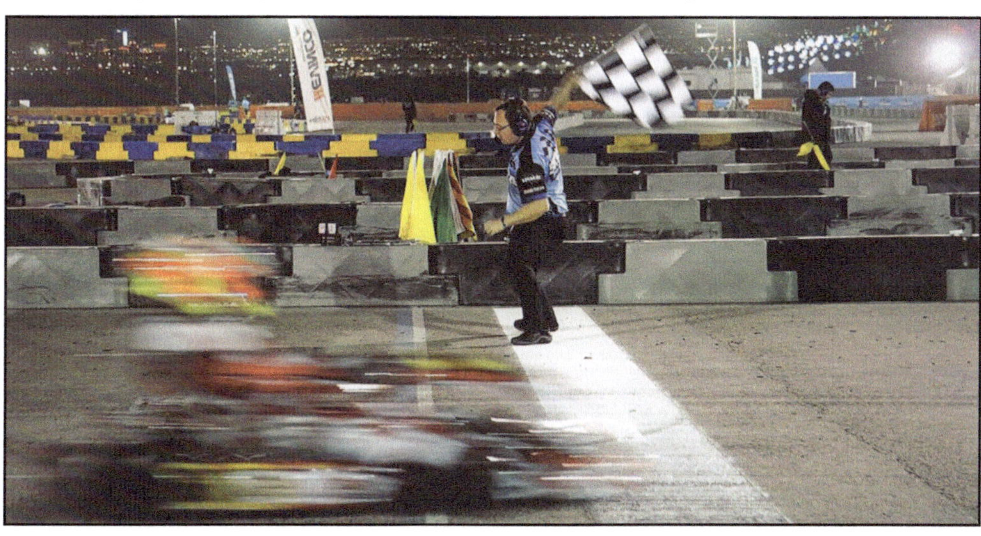

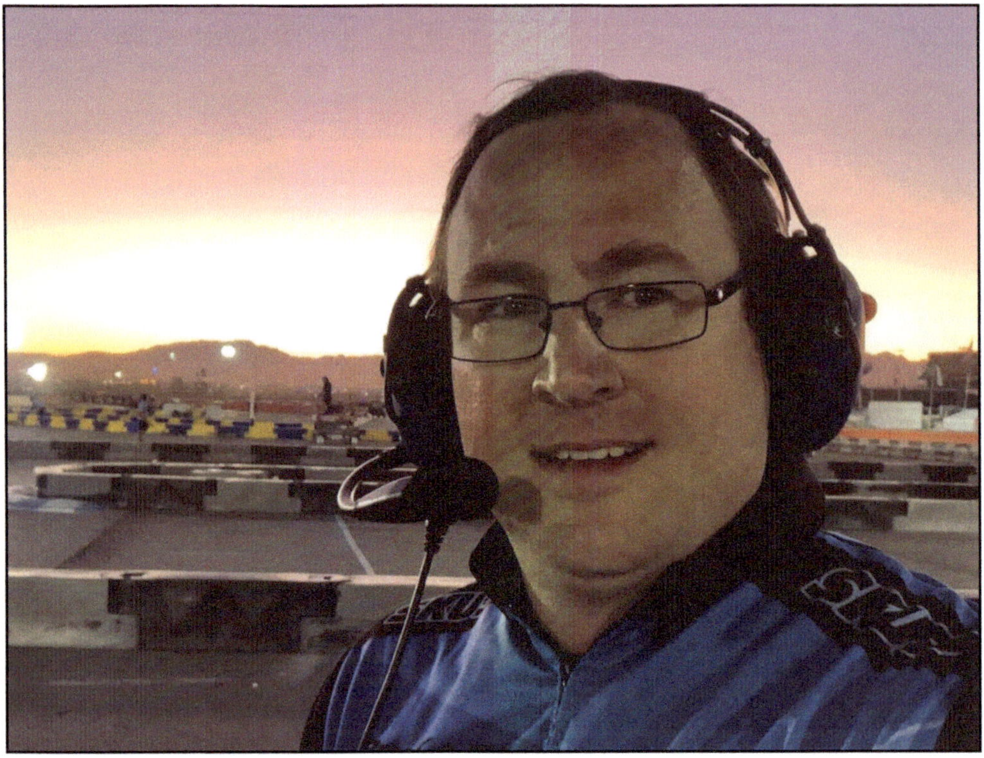

Above: Sunrise at the SKUSA SuperNationals kart race in Las Vegas.

Below: Aaron giving double checkers at the Streets of Lancaster Grand Prix, Lancaster, CA. *(On-Track Productions Photo)*

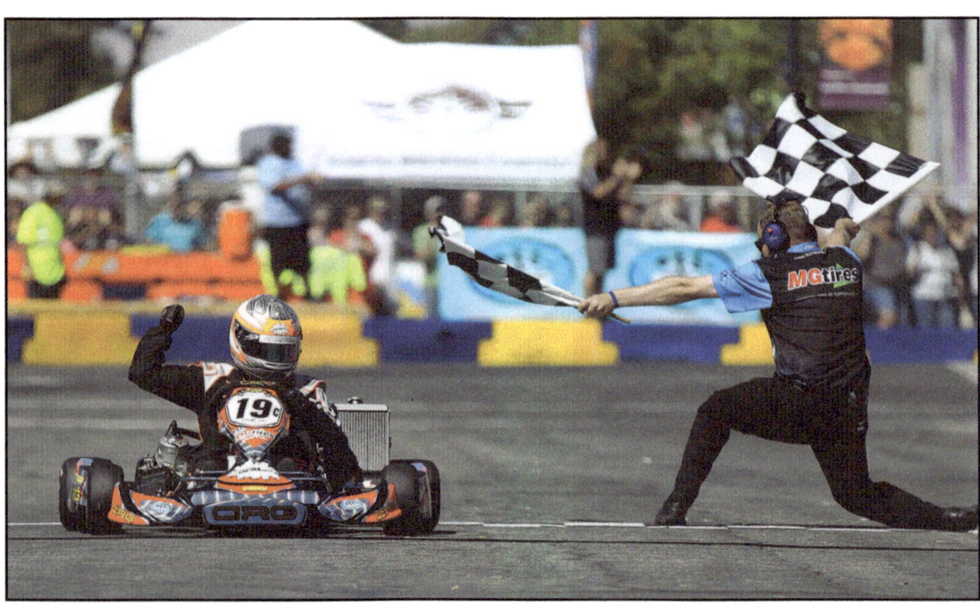

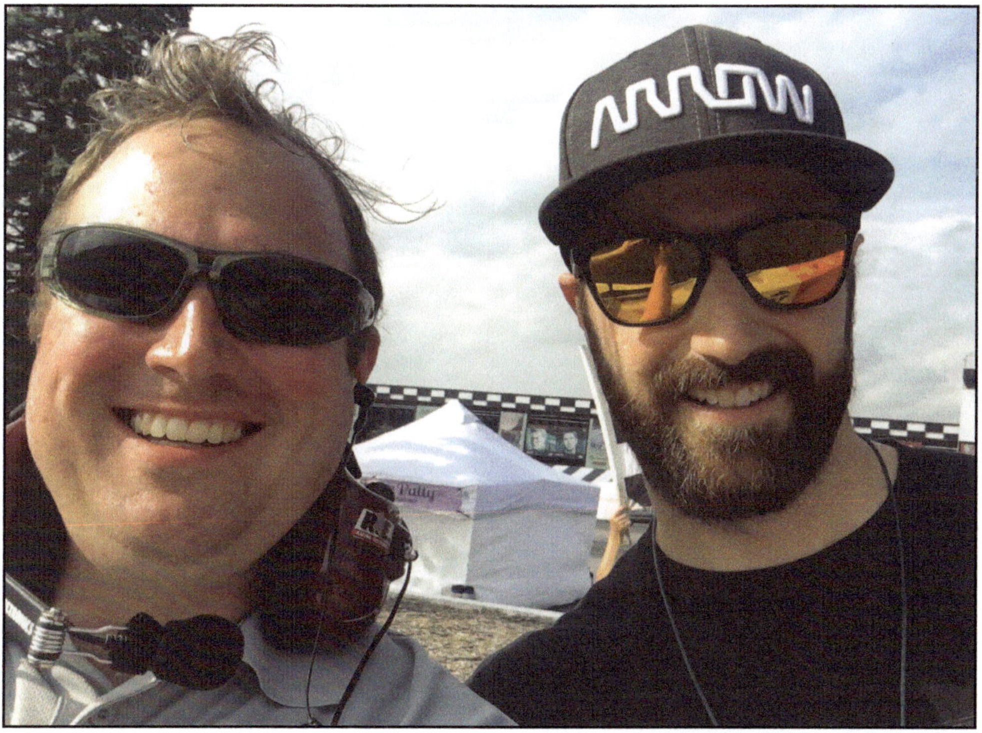

Above: James Hinchcliffe,
NBC IndyCar broadcaster
and former IndyCar driver,
was an honorary .25 Midget
flagman with Aaron in
2018.

Right: Flagging the
Battle at the Brickyard
for USAC's .25 Midget
series.

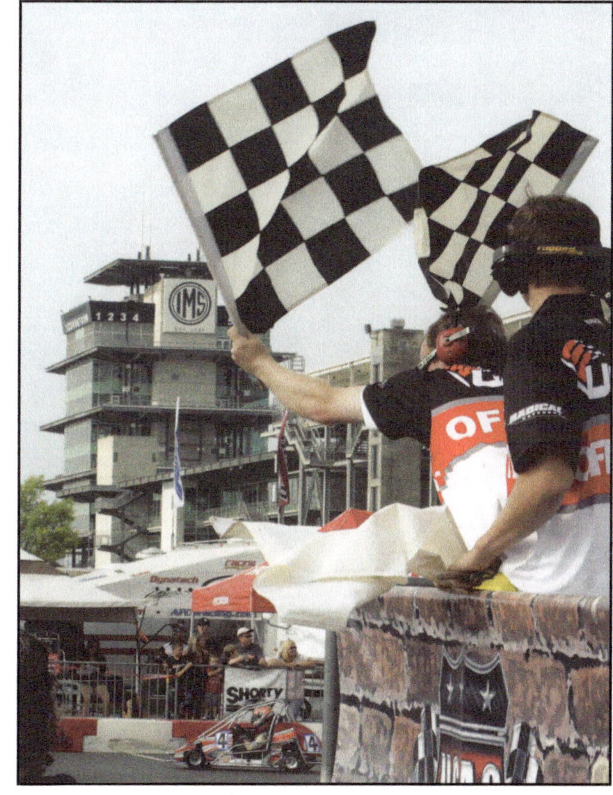

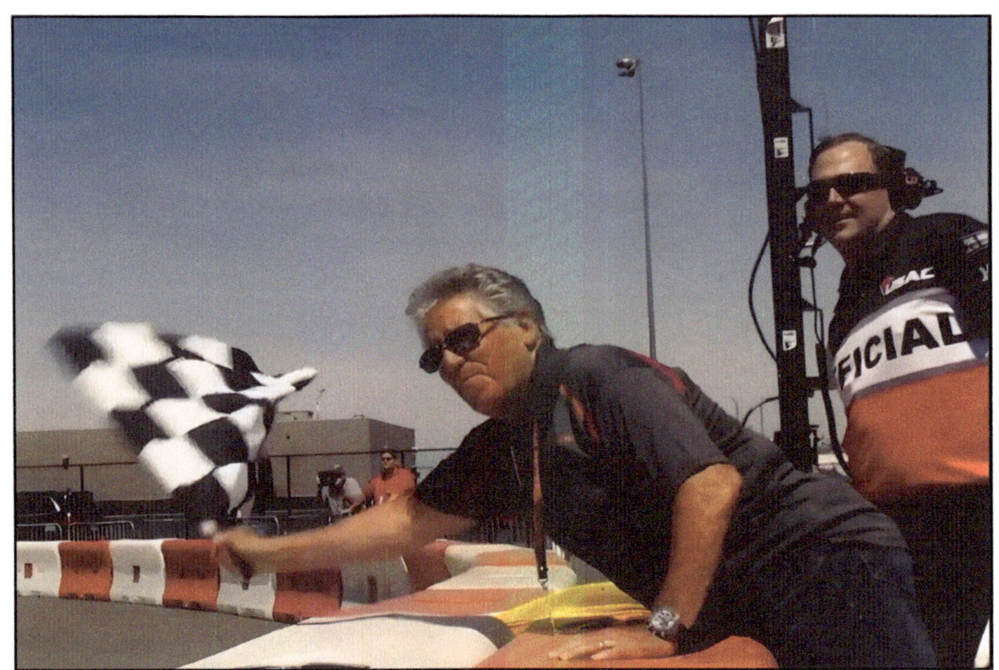

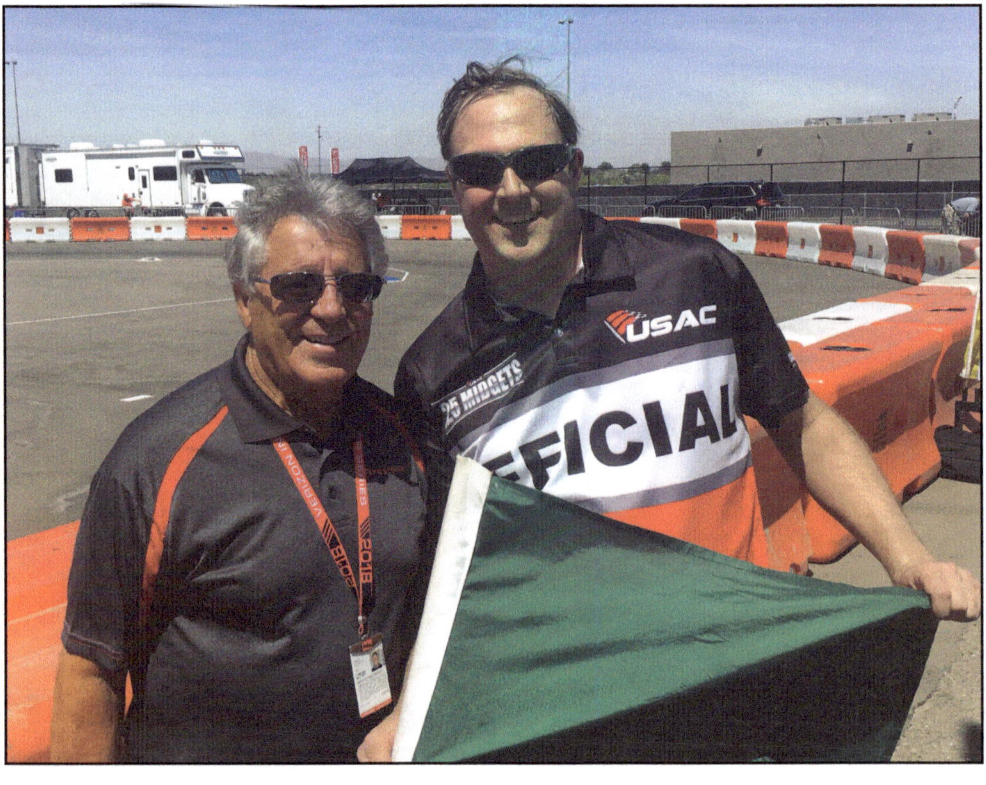

Mario Andretti served as honorary starter for a USAC .25 Midget race at Phoenix. Says Aaron, "You should know that the man can flag!"

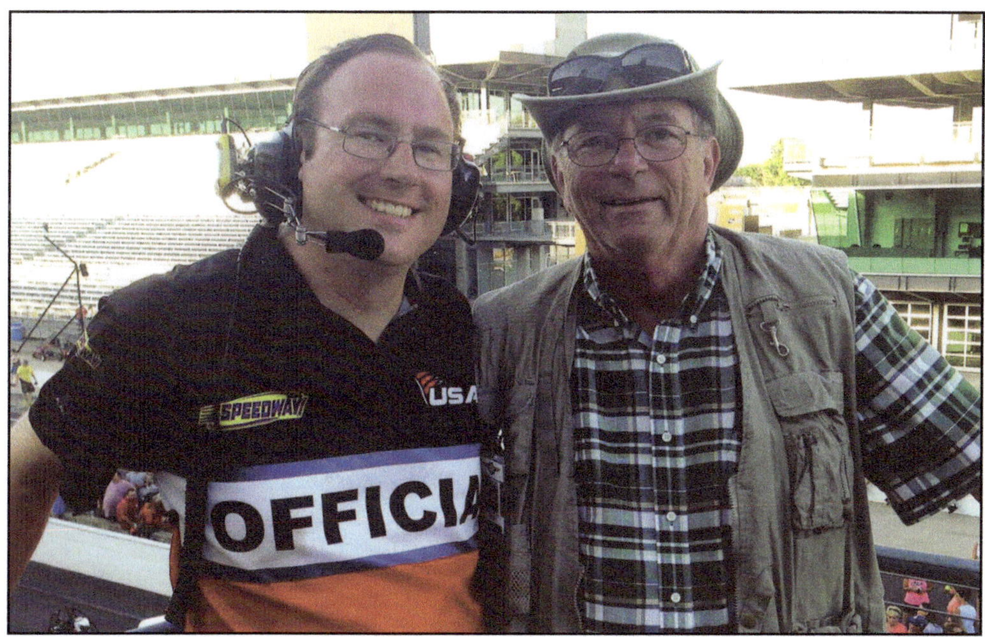

Above: Family ties—Aaron and his dad, Jim Likens, in the Indianapolis Motor Speedway flagstand.

Below: Aaron, Jeffrey "Judge" Boles, and Andrew Kremer, May 2016, Aaron's first day flagging in the IMS flagstand. *(Doug Boles Photo)*

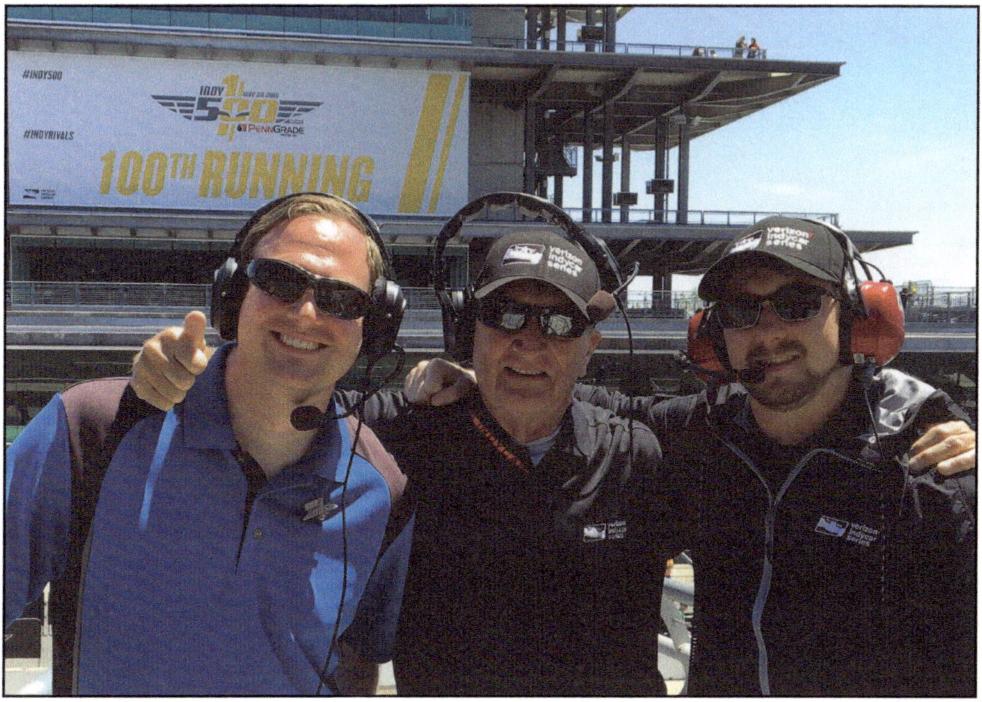

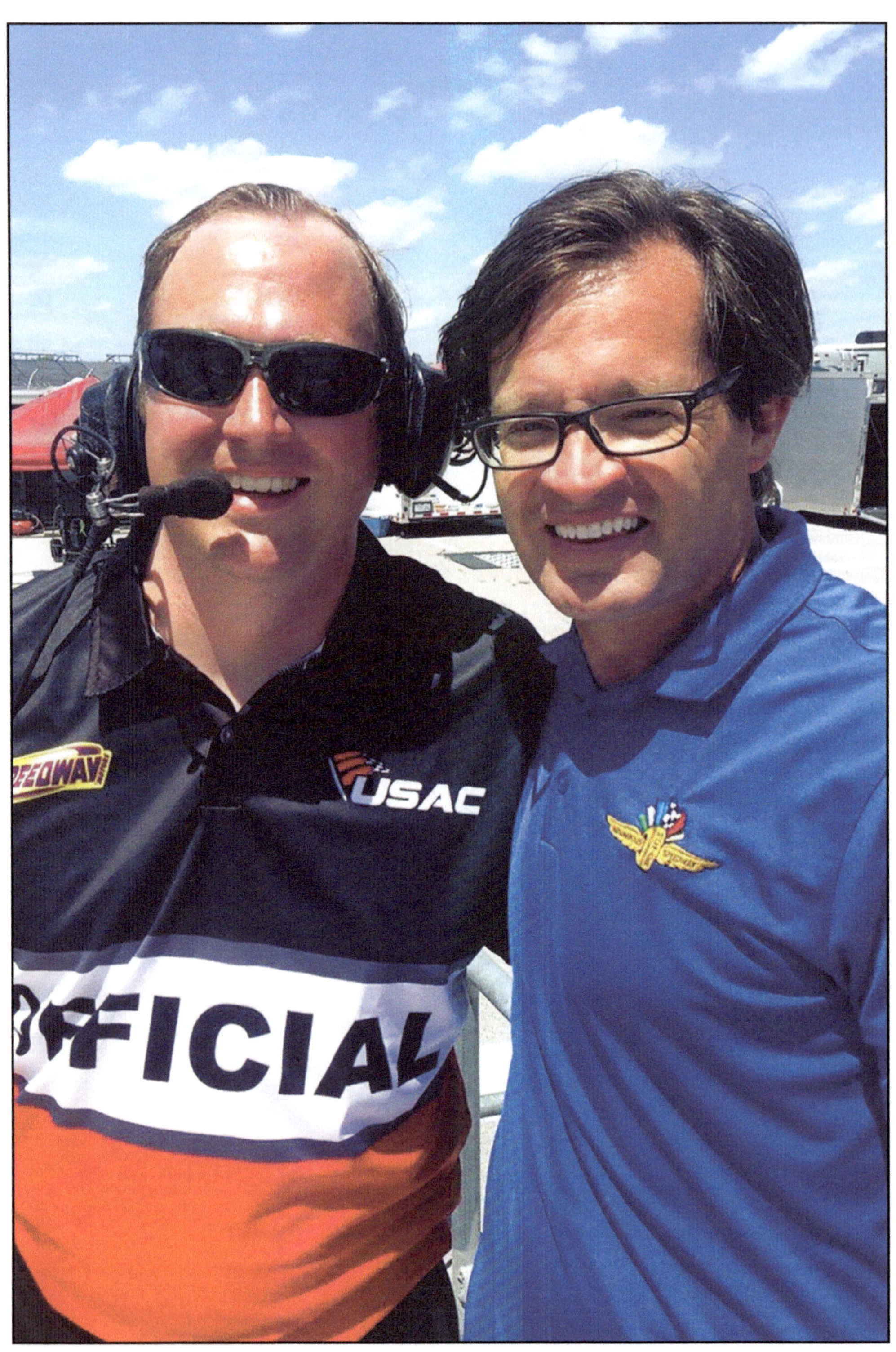

Aaron with Indianapolis Motor Speedway president Doug Boles.

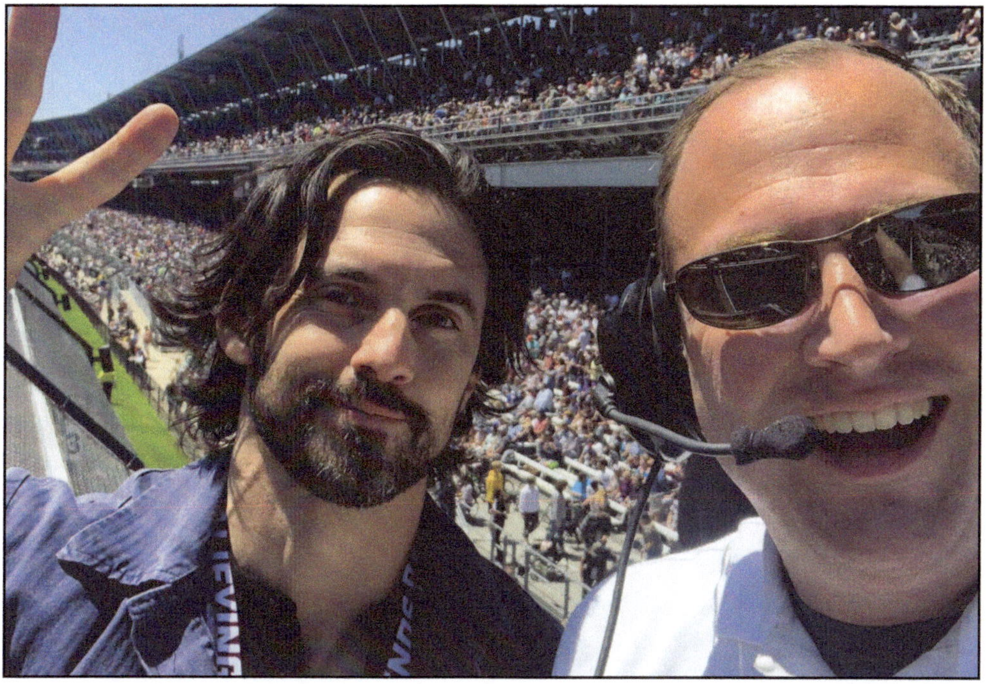

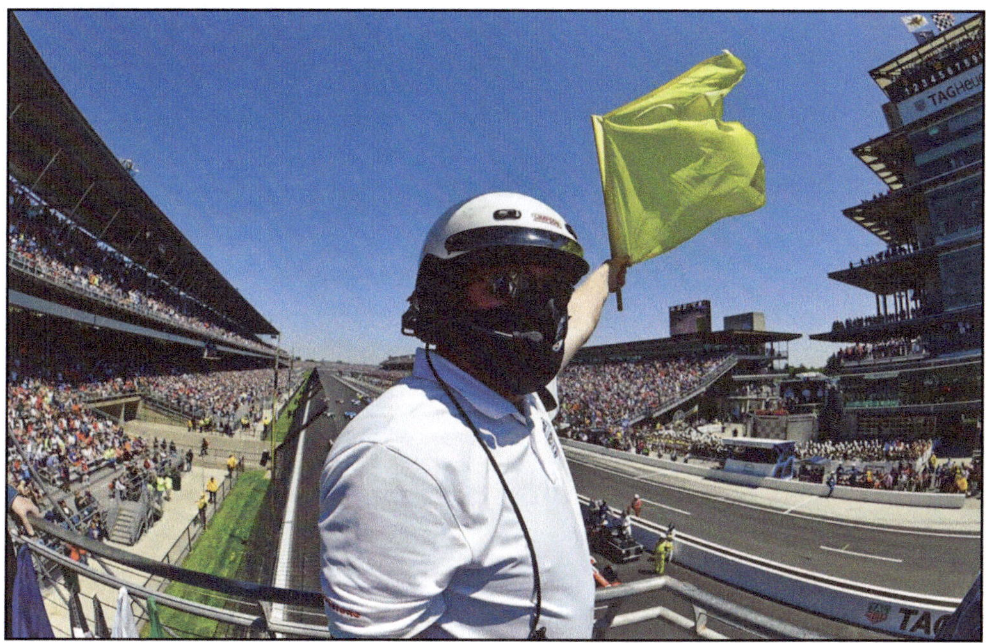

Above: Two men sharing the pre-race buzz at the 2021 Indianapolis 500. Aaron grabs a last-minute selfie with honorary starter Milo Ventimiglia.

Below: Aaron displays the yellow flag as the field rolls off prior to the 2021 Indy 500. *(Walter Kuhn Photo, IMS)*

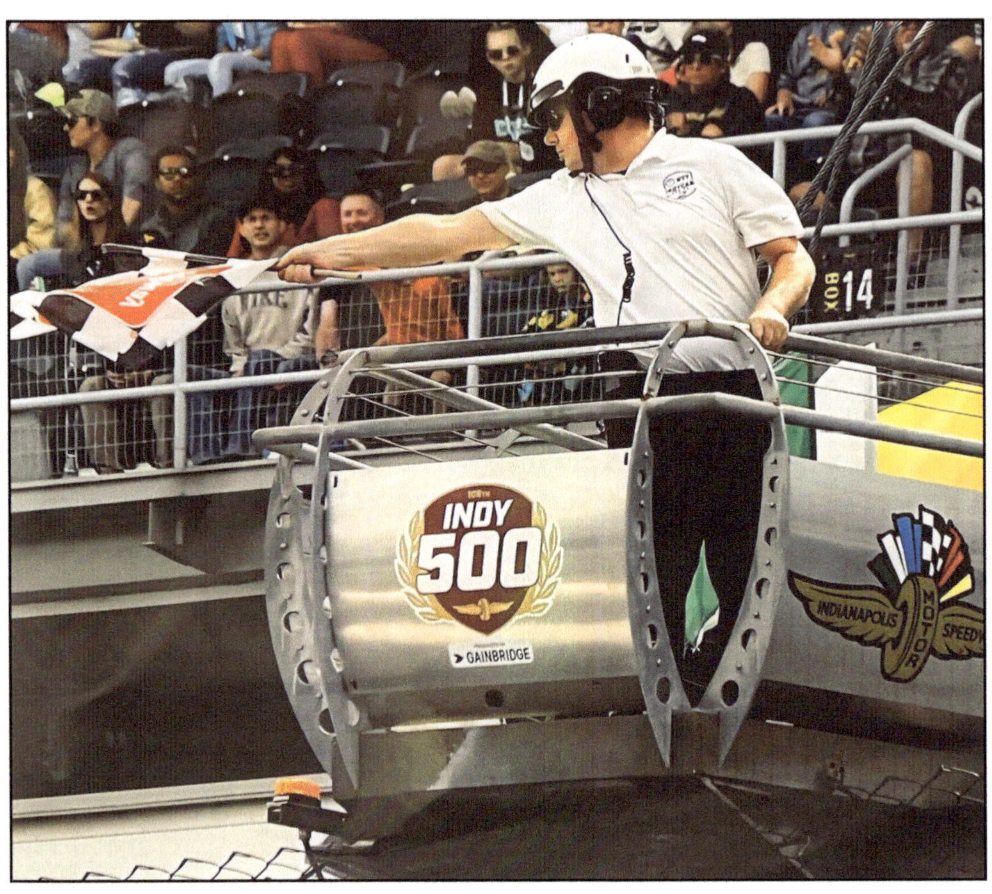

Aaron's unique point-and-freeze at the end of an Indy 500 qualifying run has become his "signature" in the eyes of many fans.

Marshalltown, Iowa, to look forward to. This meant another drive with Greg and Gary, along with Greg's dog, Annie. With each trip, I was more social; I looked forward to the journey as much as the race itself.

On practice-and-qualification day, I was informed by the track owner that the longtime flagman there would be doing the next day's races. At first, I wanted to protest this decision, but I thought back to Frankie Neidenbach and how he probably would have given anything to flag one more race. Marshalltown hadn't hosted a traveling series in a couple of years, so this was going to be a treat for him. As for me, by not flagging I could roam the track and observe things as a race director, and also be on the lookout for wildlife; in practice, I had to throw the red flag for a herd of deer running down the back straightaway. Again, just when you think you've seen it all.

Outside of being told I wasn't flagging, it was a routine weekend. Well, except for the written protest I got on a paper towel; I still have that protest to this day.

That weekend, Greg offered me a chance to go to the upcoming Rock Island Grand Prix, a street race in Rock Island, Illinois. That event had been run since 1994 and was one of American karting's premier shows. Greg needed help with bookkeeping and photography; he knew that I had some photographic experience and thought that providing photos to his karting customers would be a good idea. That worked out well, because at Rock Island I discovered an ability to take action shots. Honestly, it came naturally to me. After scoping out the track, I had a feel for where the hot spots would be, and my photos got rave reviews.

Driving back to St. Louis, Greg asked if I wanted to photograph his team at the SuperNationals in Las Vegas, the number one kart race in the world, organized by Super-Karts USA, or SKUSA. I jumped at the opportunity, and in November I rode west with Greg and Gary. The trip had a rough start, with a flat tire before we even got out of town and later a wheel flying off the trailer. This made the long drive to Vegas even longer, but I savored every minute.

I was in awe of the *size* of what everyone calls "the SuperNats." I'd never seen an international-level karting event, and this one was top-notch in all regards. I was making good money taking photos, but I was a bit envious of the flagger. I couldn't imagine the thrill of working such a prestigious event, with so many countries represented. I made it a point to stop hanging around the flagger and focus on my real responsibility.

As with Rock Island, my photos were a hit, and I helped Greg with some bookkeeping. After the SuperNats, he asked if I'd like to work part-time in his office. I said yes, so after a few days to decompress once we got home to St. Louis, I reported to PG Racing for inventory duty. Early on, I wondered if I'd bit off more than I could chew because PG had become an outlet for a popular Italian chassis, Wildkart, which might mean adding about a thousand new parts to our QuickBooks system. I later learned that most of the parts I worried about were for classes we don't run in America. Anyway, I liked the job.

In December of '06, I was invited to Greg's house for a Christmas party. Most of the team would be there. I was told to bring my flags, so I did, although I thought it was a bit odd, since this home was in an upper-middle-class neighborhood in a heavily suburban environment.

The flags did not remain a mystery for long. As I was cleaning up in my second poker tournament of the night, I heard engines in the backyard. Greg came in and told me to grab my flags, so I got them from the car and met him in the backyard. I was thrilled, and slightly concerned, about what I saw: a bright floodlight shining on a handful of pit bikes, which are essentially miniature motorcycles. The plan was to race these bikes around the trees in Greg's backyard and I would be the flagger. I was apprehensive. I mean, what would the neighbors think? It was now pushing 10:30 p.m., and I was sure they were not accustomed to late-night motorcycle races. But I succumbed to peer pressure and took my place at the start/finish line.

After warmups, just as we were set to start the first heat race, the neighbor with the yard parallel to the "backstretch" came over to say that his daughters were crying because Greg's yard was being destroyed. True, it was becoming a rutted dirt track, but that didn't stop the action. The neighbor kept an eye on us, and it definitely caught his attention when one of the racers lost control entering "turn one" and went through a fence.

It wasn't *his* fence, but the neighbor shouted, "That's it, I'm calling the cops!"

We expedited the remainder of the Christmas Party Super-Moto and finished before the police showed up on what had to be the oddest call they'd ever received from that neighborhood. There were ruts and dirt everywhere, but no pit bikes circulating, so the officers politely said, "Just make sure there's no more motorsports activity here tonight, or in the future, please."

That closed out 2006, a pretty good year. I had a job, and I was part of a team, even with my shyness and quirks. And as December ended, I'd also completed all the chapters in this project I called "Finding Kansas." It was time do something with it. Could it actually be a book?

Racing and Politics

A QUOTE LONG ATTRIBUTED TO DUANE SWEENEY GOES something like this: "So long as your love of racing exceeds your distaste of politics, you'll remain in the sport." I never fully understood what this meant until 2007, when karting-club politics in St. Louis got ugly.

Before the first wheel turned in the spring, some folks in the series tried to get rid of me as race director by finding a tax law that may have forbidden me to be paid for flagging as I was a member of the board. Whether this was a legitimate law didn't matter; what mattered was that those people knew this was an income stream for me, and they took it away.

Why did they come after me? Well, since I now worked at Greg's kart shop, the racers who shopped elsewhere thought there might be some "home cooking" when it came to the decisions I made. In other words, they were worried that I'd play favorites. This troubled me, because the thing I cared about most was the rules, and fairness. To have people who knew me thinking this way hurt me deeply.

Things only got worse from there. We had one young racer, nine or 10, who had phenomenal speed and was always a contender for the win. The problem was that with his natural speed came an extreme sense of aggression. Three-time F1 World Champion Ayrton Senna famously said, "If you no longer go for a gap that exists, you're no longer a racing driver." Well, this kid made his own gaps, and by any means necessary. He was becoming dangerous. In the previous season I'd had conversations with him, as had several members of the board, about tempering that aggression. We were hoping to head off the possibility of a nasty crash.

There's a fine balance between tapering excessive aggression and negatively influencing speed. I didn't want to do anything that might hinder his development as a driver, or as a kid. At the same time, the race director has a responsibility for everyone's safety. Well, as the green flag dropped in one event, he attempted to go from seventh to first with a four-wide pass. Instead, he launched over a curb and landed on the shoulder of another racer. Something had to be done.

The next time around, I gave him a furled black flag. This was not a warning. I had seen enough. I also mentioned to the club president and vice president that while I hadn't made up my mind, I was considering an event disqualification, which would exclude him from the day's final.

During the lunch break, I had made my decision: the kid would not be allowed to race that afternoon. The club president tried to talk me out of it, in a gentle, club-politics way, but my stance was that if this level of disregard for others continued, we might see a hideous crash; I added that we were lucky not to have had a hideous result from his first incident.

The president, vice president, and I walked to his pit area. As we got there, the kid's dad began knocking stuff around and said, "We're going home! They don't want us here!" I hated this kind of thing. Why did I accept this level of responsibility? Like a stone tumbling down a steep hill, we could not slow down the scene that was unfolding. We tried to use reason but were met with anger. The dad mentioned other incidents and crashes that didn't result in event disqualifications, and I kept replying that none of those other drivers had a yearlong record of repeated issues. After a couple minutes of failed diplomacy, the parent demanded that I talk with his son, and I had no problem doing that.

The kid exited the trailer in tears; he had heard our debate with his dad. It was all on me now. I didn't want to destroy the kid. I talked about his future and his incredible speed and said that I was sure he didn't want to hurt anyone. But I added that racing can be dangerous, and that in my opinion his moves exceeded acceptable risk. I told him that with his raw talent, he could have a long career in racing. I said that I knew that watching the final, rather than racing in it, was going to hurt, but I hoped he would think about the need to finish races without knocking people off the track.

He took it better than his dad, even though he was crying. When the conversation was over, I, too, was almost in tears. Thankfully, I never had to have that conversation with him again, and he quickly developed an ability to pass others without contact.

I thought I handled the situation gracefully, and I was elated that the social aspect of it didn't overwhelm me. Conflict had been something I had avoided at all costs in my life, but "playing" the role of race director—much as an actor plays a role on stage—allowed me to handle it without fear. Conflict was not something to be feared, but rather something to be listened to, mitigated, and adjudicated by me.

The following weekend, I made note of several jump-start penalties in the heat races. Per the rulebook, I had the final say in all penalties. The process was simple: I would radio the scorers, they would log it, and the penalty would be given at the scales. I was unaware that a club official that day had been overriding my penalties, which he didn't have the authority to do. When it came time for the main events, I noticed that the penalties I'd assessed had not taken effect. I got on the radio and asked what had happened. The person who had issued the vetoes said, "Aaron, those penalties were unfair. You can't be biased."

Well, there had *been* no bias. The cruel thing known as club politics had come into play. This person was affiliated with "the other kart shop," and I was in the middle of a shop war that didn't actually exist; neither of the shop owners was waging war, but it was their customers who thought a war was going on. Now the race director's authority had been torn down—whether the director was me, or anyone else—and my own impartiality had been attacked. The terms "unfair" and "you can't be biased" tore through my skull like cannonballs through a ship's hull.

Did I handle this with the grace and poise I'd shown the previous week after barring that kid from the final? Did I handle it as calmly as I handled those three-wide situations as a driver? No. I simply stopped talking. That was always the first step in my descents into darkness.

There's a misconception that those on the autism spectrum have fewer emotions than "normal" people. For some, this may be true, but my version is that I won't *show* my emotions. And kept inside, they can be overwhelming. Biased and unfair? My emotions were off the chart as I dealt with those accusations.

I should've fired back my reasoning for the penalties, but I didn't. As the minutes went on, I was a mess, trapped in my own thoughts. All the while, I'm doing my job, flagging the races, even as every nerve in my body hurt with this emotional rage that had nowhere to go.

I made it through the day. Later, as the board members who were on my side—and there should have been no "sides," only a single board—went through the events of the day, they identified the mistakes that had been made, and the person who had been vetoing my on-track calls apologized. I realized that I would have to be stronger as a person should something like this happen again.

I thought a lot about Duane Sweeney's quote: "So long as your love of racing exceeds your distaste of politics, you'll remain in the sport." And I remained in the sport.

Back Behind the Wheel

MY DAD STARTED HANDLING GREG'S PG RACING WEBSITE, and as a trade-out I'd get to drive in some of the non-CSSS races that Greg's team went to. Most of these were on road courses, longer than those where karts typically run. I'd be at these events anyway, helping with the bookkeeping and accepting payments for the shop, but now I'd also be racing once again.

I had dreams of running for a championship, but I quickly realized that my equipment wasn't a priority. Besides, the road-racing grids were set by the postmark on the entry payment, and by not pre-entering, I'd always be starting last. Also, if one of the primary team racers had issues, "my" kart would likely be available to them. It was hard to rationalize racing with having almost no chance of winning, but I did my best.

My favorite part of these events, as had become the norm, was the travel. Whether we went to Road America, GingerMan, or Grattan Raceway Park in Belding, Michigan, the travel made me feel free. On the other hand, the racing itself could sometimes get aggravating.

Perhaps every racer has had a weekend like I did at Road America in 2007, but in five on-track sessions, only once did I make it more than a lap. The other four times, I broke down somewhere. I did get to see the track from some of Road America's signature locations, like beneath the Sargento Bridge or outside Canada Corner, but with each mechanical failure I was relegated to watching other people have fun out on the track, which ate at me.

The road-racing series then went to Grattan Raceway Park, where the only ride available to me was a shifter kart. I protested that I had never raced one of those. Speeds in shifter karts can easily reach triple digits, and at this track there was a spot where a kart would actually go airborne over a crest. There wasn't really any room for doubting one's skill, and I doubted mine.

The kart I was in had a lesser engine than the others in the class, but I had only two choices: accept the slow kart, or don't race. Most of the teams competing for the win were Greg's customers, and I didn't want to get in their way—or anyone else's—when I inevitably got lapped. Before the race, I implored Greg to signal to me when the leaders were coming behind me.

I had never used a hand clutch before, and I went into the race knowing that just like in the formula cars I'd driven at the Derek Daly Academy, shifting was not my strong suit.

So, there I was, already off-pace thanks to my engine, and now having to manage shifting gears on a big road course with serious elevation changes, and, by the way, a pack of a dozen karts battling for the win. I knew they would at some point swallow me up and perhaps even pass me on both sides. This was going to be a disaster.

On each lap, I'd spot Greg on the pit wall and await a signal of some sort. We'd never established what type of signal it would be, but I looked anyway. Finally, about three-quarters of the way through the race, he pointed up and then behind me. The leaders were coming. I didn't want to influence the race; these were Greg's customers, and any misjudgment by me could hurt his business. The stakes were high.

That lap, as I approached the crest I mentioned earlier, I glanced behind me and saw a train of karts closing. I panicked. As I refocused forward, I hit the crest off-center, which put my kart sideways over the jump. When I landed, my front wheels were pointed to the left, so my kart turned hard in that direction. I ran off the track, down the hill, and into weeds that stood taller than I did. As at Road America, I had an interesting viewpoint to watch the rest of the race.

There in the weeds, I had this thought for the first time: "I don't need this in my life. Why am I doing this?" But it went away quickly. There was, however, that one question that never seemed to go away: "What am I going to do with my life?"

A Crash in Marshalltown

IT WAS NOW PAST THE MID-SEASON MARK, AND LIFE HAD settled into a stagnant groove. I worked during the week, played Xbox when home, and looked forward to the next race weekend. I did some occasional writing, but for the most part I avoided thinking about that troubling question about the rest of my life, and what to do with it.

The next race on the CSSS schedule was Marshalltown, where the previous year I'd surrendered my flagging duties to the local starter. This time, I'd have the position.

It was so hot that weekend in the middle of Iowa that I didn't really want to take my usual track walk, but I did any-way. At the next-to-last corner, a steeply banked hairpin—it reminded me of a cereal bowl—I saw that the fence had no protection at its exit. The year prior, it had been lined with the type of Tecpro barriers you often see at Formula 1 races. As I gazed over the lip of the bowl, there was a narrow strip of grass, then what's called a hog fence, thick wire in a wood frame, and lastly a chain-link fence. I could see the Tecpros; they were stacked up in the parking lot. I talked to Greg, then with the track owners, who said, "Don't worry about that. No one's ever gone into that fence since it's such a slow-speed corner." As I opened my mouth to lobby for the Tecpro, the owner said again, "Aaron, don't worry about it."

This was the middle of the 2007 CSSS season, and I was loving it because in this series, there was no politics. I got paid to direct and flag. But on this weekend, if it looked like the final in the senior class was going to be a runaway, I was going to hop into a kart and race. Looking back, I laugh about racing *and* being race director. But the Marshalltown track was a blast, and I wanted all the seat time I could get.

Indeed, it looked as if everyone was going to behave themselves, so for the final I hopped into a kart and started last. I had a great start, and considering that I had no practice, I was doing well, staying with the pack. I wasn't going to fool myself into thinking I had a shot at a great finish; many of the drivers in front of me were national-caliber drivers. I just wanted to do the best I could and enjoy the amazing speed of these karts.

I was absolutely hounding the kart in front of me, but Marshalltown was on the narrow side. Try as I might, I could not get alongside this driver. Sure, I could have dive-bombed him, but why? I wasn't racing for anything but fun, so it didn't matter if I was ninth, 10th, or 16th.

Being so focused on that kart, I pushed aside an odd sensation I was feeling as I entered the corners. There was a delay when I applied the brakes; not much, but enough that I should've considered that it might be a developing issue. Yeah, so much for being in this for fun; I wanted this pass! Entering turn four, I overshot the corner and almost hit the rear bumper of the kart just ahead. I wondered how I could make such a silly error. Little did I know that it wasn't me.

Earlier, at my driver's meeting, I mentioned that we hadn't had any red flags, and I wanted it to stay that way. I said, "Don't be the red flag this weekend!" I had that flash-back as I came so close to the kart in front of me. But now, through the switchback of turn five, setting up for the two corners leading into the cereal bowl, I focused, ready to make my move.

Headed into the banking, I put my foot on the brake … and there was *nothing*. The kart in front of me slowed for the corner, and I was closing at an alarming speed. To miss him, I turned into the bowl early. I went past him, but with my speed there was no way to make the corner.

My sudden flick of the wheel put me into a slide, and I was sideways in this banked, bowl-like turn. Time seemed to speed up. I slid over the lip of the banking and got air-borne, headed straight for that unprotected hog fence. I saw it coming, and knew I was in trouble.

You've heard that cliché where people say that in moments of great danger, their lives flashed before their eyes? Believe it, because it happened to me. Years and years of thoughts, in less than a second, including this: "So I'm about to die. Has everything been for nothing?" This was the depth of my thinking, even in this crash; I regretted much of my life, the bits that autism hindered. I regretted the experiences I *didn't* have, the ones I knew everyone else had.

That hog fence terrified me. I thought that if I hit it the wrong way, I might lose an arm, as gruesome as that sounds. I lowered my head and prayed. The fence *devoured* the kart. My body hit it first with my right shin; the fence then smashed my hand where my fingers wrapped around the steering wheel. My head impacted the frame of the fence, and I blacked out briefly.

When I came to, I could see Greg waving the red flag from the starter's stand. I was confused; why was *he* flagging? I saw a couple kids sprinting towards me. Why were they running? I tried to look up, then I realized that I couldn't because I was wrapped up in the fence. I tried to take a breath, and all I felt was pain.

The barrier I'd asked for would've prevented this crash from reaching this level. I'd have been stopped by the Tecpro, and not crashed through the fencing. The cross beam of the hog fence rested against the lip of my helmet; wait, it wasn't *my* helmet. My helmet was back in St. Louis, and Greg had lent me his, which had an extended lip at the bottom. It was that lip that prevented my throat from hitting the cross bar. Had that happened, well, I doubt you'd be reading this.

The track ambulance personnel called the fire department to carefully extricate me. Fencing had to be cut, and because witnesses told the paramedics how much my neck had twisted in the impact, every precaution was taken.

I was unable to provide much verbal feedback on how I felt, and for that I would blame the concussive blow to my helmet. I do remember being placed in a special harness that lifted me straight out of the kart, and then I was placed on a backboard and rushed to the hospital.

As much as the crash hurt, the discomfort in the emergency room was close to the same level. I was still strapped down on the backboard, with the helmet on. My suit—also borrowed from Greg—had been cut off of me. I wondered if Greg would be mad, losing a kart *and* a suit.

The thoughts of regret I'd had just before hitting the fence crept back in, and I let out a mighty sigh. It was then that I could hear someone else in the room; seated in the corner was the mom of one of the younger racers, sent by Greg to be with me. She asked what hurt, and I said it would be easier to list what *didn't* hurt. A doctor came in and asked what happened. I hoped the mom might answer for me because I was still confused. I remembered the trip into the fence, and the horrible thoughts of all the things I should've done in my life. But what *had* happened?

The mom said, "Aaron was racing a kart. The starter battery became dislodged, and it slowly cut the brake line until there was no fluid left." That was the answer. Brake failure.

Next came a couple of hours of tests and being maneuvered around like a square log because I was still strapped down. I felt as if blood was pooling in the back of my head from the helmet being tied down. I started crying the deepest, most mournful tears of my life. They weren't tears from physical pain, but from a pain rooted at the level of the soul. Why was everything so hard? Why wasn't I fulfilling what I felt I was put on Earth to do? I shouldn't be hitting fences in Iowa; I should've been taking checkered flags at Daytona, Monza, Spa, or, preferably, Indianapolis. Yet there I was, tied down on my back and in immense pain.

"God hates me!" I exclaimed.

The mom was taken aback, and asked how I came to that conclusion. This froze me. I was expecting her to reply,

"No, that's not true," but instead she asked a logical question. I began laying out my case, which temporarily helped me overlook the pain.

As I went on, the doctor came in. All the tests for a broken neck were negative, so the helmet came off. The mom had started her rebuttal, saying that everything happens to put us where we need to be, and nothing happens by accident. Of course, I *knew* this; remember, my dad is a pastor. But when the doctor looked over the helmet and mentioned that the extended chin area probably prevented worse injury, the mom responded, "See? My point is proven."

The crash left me with a strained neck, a concussion, some brutally swollen fingers, and a hematoma on each of my shins. It was a long ride back to St. Louis the following day. Greg was already talking about getting me into a kart again. I wanted that, too; I didn't want the fear of crashing to end my love of driving.

A month later, at 61 Kartway in Delmar, Iowa, I drove some practice laps, just to shake off the cobwebs. There was no fear.

After I returned to race-director duty, the son of Greg's girlfriend ran up and asked, "Did you see that kart fly?"

I was confused. Then another kart stopped at the pit exit, where I was standing, and the driver was screaming. Something awful had happened.

This track had some extreme elevation changes and an amazing horseshoe corner. Greg's lead driver's girlfriend was driving the kart I'd been on. A nut became dislodged and stuck in the carburetor, hanging the throttle open. She went into that horseshoe corner at full speed, then up a steep hill; the kart flew some 150 feet before landing. She suffered some nasty hip injuries.

Once we knew that she was going to be fine, it occurred to me how lucky I was not to be in that kart. The mom who had been with me in the hospital found me and said, "See?

God has a reason he kept you safe through those two events. Just wait."

I'd *been* waiting. But waiting for what?

── **Reaching the Top Amid Darkness** ──

AS 2007 DREW TO AN END, POLITICS CONTINUED TO PLAGUE the St. Louis Karting Association. There were disagreements over racing technology, and it was clear that the new board of directors looked vindictively toward the previous board. I was advised to not stay on as the SKLA flagger, but that was something I'd done since 1995. How could I just let that go? The six CSSS races per season were not enough to keep me motivated.

But right from the very first race of '08, this wasn't the SLKA I knew. A couple of years earlier, we were north of 150 karts at some meets; now there were just 40. It was strange that despite the obvious evidence that the club was dying, those who remained had almost a celebratory air about them. They were in control, they were getting what *they* wanted, so they were happy. They were like the victors of a nuclear war, surrounded by complete destruction but unable to see it because *they* had survived. It made no sense to me. It was hard to put my normal energy into flagging races with as few as two karts.

The following week I wrote an email indicating that I was stepping down as SLKA flagman. In my time with the club, I had missed only two races, one in 2000 when I was in Alaska and the other in '03 when I was in Las Vegas. It felt as if a part of my life was dying. I sobbed as the mouse icon hovered over the "send" button; this was an email I would not be able to take back. Could I throw away 12 years with one click of a mouse? I don't like change, but finally I decided that this change was right. I sent the email and said goodbye to the St. Louis Karting Association.

Interestingly, the first CSSS race of the season was set to be on SLKA turf, at the I-55 Speedway karting circuit in Pevely, Missouri. The series was now affiliated with SKUSA and renamed the SKUSA Central States Challenge. SKUSA president Tom Kutscher came to St. Louis to kick off the new regional series, which added a bit of pressure for me. As race director and flagger, I wanted things to be perfect.

That weekend started off smoothly, with no issues on track. Being a race director would be such an easy job if every weekend went like that. The series had rented the track, so it was our show, and the kart club didn't have any say in what took place. It felt like an SLKA event from previous years; all the teams fed up with the politics came back to race.

I felt a lot of joy. As I displayed the final double checkered of the weekend, I teared up; this was probably going to be my last race flagging with a lot of people I had known for years. Letting go of SKLA meant also letting go, to some degree, of my memories of flagging with Frankie Neidenbach, and all the joys and challenges that had made me who I was. It was emotional for me, and I think that added some extra flair to my flagging.

One of the race director's jobs is to deal with post-race protests. As soon as I was certain there were none, I headed for my car, still full of emotion. Greg Yocom stopped me and said that I was needed at the podium ceremony. There's no arguing with the boss, so I walked over and stood by the podium, still teary behind my sunglasses.

The trophies were just about all handed out, and I was still standing around. Why was I there? I recall thinking that I could have been home already. Driving away immediately would have been like ripping the emotional band-aid straight off, getting it over with.

Before the final class was called, SKUSA's Tom Kutscher took the microphone. I was staring off towards the property exit, but I did hear Tom say, in a serious tone, "Okay, folks, I've been to many tracks, but I've never seen the shit I saw this weekend."

Oh, man. What the hell? This was bad. This was very bad. Had I done something wrong? I couldn't think of anything. But I was frozen, awaiting a punch in the face.

"Yes, folks," Tom continued, "I've been to many tracks all over the world and I've never seen what I saw today. And that leaves me with just one question …"

Time froze. Was this not only the end of my time in St. Louis, but racing in general? I didn't know if his words were directed my way, but I worried that they were.

"Aaron …"

No, no, no. No! This was the end, I was sure.

"I just want to say I have found my new flagger for the SKUSA SuperNats. Do you want the job?"

What? I'm sure I was staring at Tom Kutscher with a blank expression. Did I hear him correctly? The SuperNats is a truly international event. NASCAR drivers, IndyCar drivers, even F1 drivers have raced in it. Did I want to be the flagger? This was like a minor league umpire being invited to work the World Series.

My tears of sadness were quickly replaced by tears of joy. I tried to vocalize a "yes," but I was frozen. I did nod, probably in an awkward way, and the crowd gathered around the podium applauded as loudly as they had for any race winner.

Leaving the property was not painful at all. I drove away celebrating. What for a while seemed like a sad day had turned into the most joyous one imaginable.

I was so elated that I didn't call my dad on the drive home. I wanted to give him the news personally. He had actually been at the race but left before the end. When I walked into the house, I was grinning from ear to ear. Perplexed, my dad simply asked, "What?"

I recounted the story of being asked to stay for the podium ceremonies, and then I started crying tears of joy again. I ended with: "I'm now the flagman for the biggest kart race in the world!"

My dad said, "Maybe this is what you've been waiting for."

Maybe it was.

Death at the Track, Death on the Road, Death in the Family, and a Horse

I'M NOT SURE EVERYONE HAS A MIDDLE SEGMENT TO THEIR story that plays out like the part of a movie where lessons are learned about the value of life, who they are, and what they want to be, but in my life, that was the summer of 2008. It started with a trip to Road America with Greg's team. I was hoping that, unlike 2007, I might get to see turn one at speed, instead of slowing down with mechanical issues.

The draft at Road America in a kart is something that I wish everyone could feel. You pull up on the kart ahead with an incredible speed difference, like something out of a video game, but when you pull out to pass you run into a wall of air. You can *feel* the slowdown in your body. It's even more fun to bump-draft: instead of passing a kart, you lock onto his rear bumper and push, and you both gain speed.

The officials decided that bump-drafting was not allowed, but all the racers knew where the officials were stationed, and they simply bump-drafted elsewhere.

In one practice session, I drove a shifter kart. The speeds were incredible, over 100 MPH, although on such a big track it didn't always seem that fast. In full-sized cars, there are many heavy-braking zones at Road America, but in karts the brake pedal wasn't used much.

Late Saturday, I was working Greg's parts trailer when a driver named Adam Schatz, one of the better road racers, rushed in. His kart wouldn't start, and he needed a part, which somehow, I found for him; I barely knew the difference between a lug nut and a wing nut. He thanked me, and as he exited the trailer, he was putting his helmet on.

I could see only part of the front straightaway from the trailer, but I spotted Greg on the pit wall, watching the class that was running its main event. Because of the drafting, kart racing at Road America is akin to NASCAR at Talladega: thrilling, but dangerous. At the moment, there was a train of karts bump-drafting. Then, with the laps winding down, I saw karts pulling into the pit lane. The red flag had come out. This wasn't the first one of the day. A couple of team members had been in a serious wreck at the notorious "kink" in a shifter-kart race. They were uninjured, but now the red flag had come out once more.

A few minutes later, one of the team's drivers came into the trailer. He looked lost. I was about to say something when he pounded the table in anger. I didn't understand what was going on, so I asked, "Everything okay?" He just pointed towards the final corner. I headed that way.

Descending the hill, I could see paramedics tending to a driver lying on the track. I recognized the suit; it was Adam Schatz. There was complete silence as the paramedics worked; they were almost mechanical in their movements. Having seen plenty of racing and too many crashes, I feared the worst. A week later, those fears were realized; Adam died from his injuries.

I regretted that I'd known where to find that part for him.

Adam's passing really impacted me. I lost any drive to be a competitor, and after that weekend I never turned another lap on a professional track.

A week later, I was driving home from Greg's new shop in Wentzville, Missouri, 35 miles west of St. Louis. Roadwork had closed I-64 from I-270, St. Louis's beltway, to downtown. This created a logjam at the exit to I-270. As I turned onto the ramp, I saw a flash in my mirror that looked like parts flying. I thought nothing of it, but that night the TV news said a distracted semi-truck driver had plowed into the line of slow cars, killing multiple drivers.

Close calls like that sometimes made me question why I was still here. Mortality was on my mind again the following weekend. The SKUSA CSC was at West Quincy, and I don't recall anything from that meet except getting a text that said my aunt Joni had died. It was unexpected, and I didn't know how to process it. I hadn't seen her in eight years, but, because I was already dealing with issues of mortality, I took great sadness from this news.

My mom and aunt lived in Rapid City, South Dakota, and I hadn't seen my mom since 2004. Early Monday morning, I hit the open road to drive out there and pay my respects. When it was finally time to head back to St. Louis, I left at 4:00 a.m. When I take major road trips, I always try to depart while it's still dark. It lessens the emotion of leaving because at that hour I'm too tired to feel much. But my mom was extremely sad that morning; to her, my leaving meant saying goodbye to another family member. I promised not to wait as long for my next visit. With many tears, I departed.

Before I'd gone 10 miles, my phone rang. It was my mom; she just needed to hear my voice a little bit more.

A car came along in the other direction, and I turned off my high beams. Moments later, just as my mom told me she loved me, I saw what looked like black specter in the night. But it wasn't a ghost, it was a *horse*. I had no time to steer around it, and besides, I didn't know what I'd hit if I did steer off the road. I let out a scream as we collided.

The horse slid up the hood and smashed the windshield. I somehow maintained control and pulled to the side of the road. I was in a state of shock, yet I realized what had happened. My mom—who had heard her son scream, heard the impact, and heard breaking glass—was still on the phone. I told her, "Mom, I hit a horse. Come get me."

She hung up, and I tried to get out of the car. The windshield was on my hands, and bits of glass peppered my face. The car's A-post had caved in a bit, but it hadn't failed. There was pain, but I climbed out and started to direct traffic; there were a few early risers already on the road, and I had to guide them around the horse.

My mom arrived, as did the police. The trooper's first question was, "Where's the body of the driver?" He didn't believe I'd been in the car until he got close and saw the glass in my skin. Next, he and another officer who'd pulled up tried to blame me for the incident. They asked if I'd been going 80 MPH; when I said it was more like 45, they asked if I had *aimed* for the horse. I pointed out that it was a black horse on a black road on a black night, and that I saw it only at the last moment. We all noticed that the gates to an adjacent field had been left open.

It had been another brush with mortality.

Things were a nightmare from there, because my insurance didn't include horse coverage —who knew?—and neither the horse's owner nor I had the means to replace my car, or even to fix it. I stayed in Rapid City a month, and in the middle of that period my mom was kind enough to take me to 61 Kartway in Iowa, a *long* drive from home for her. It was quite a trip; this was the first time in a long while that she saw me work a race, and her little Yorkie dog bit the track owner's son; my mom said he deserved it. It was good to reconnect with her after so long.

When it came time for me to leave Rapid City a second time, there were no incidents with horses or anything else. That summer of '08 changed me. It was difficult letting go of my dream of being a championship-caliber racer, but I liked working as an official. And maybe something good would happen with my book; I was now just a month away from receiving the self-published version. Whatever was ahead, I thanked God for seeing me through so many dramatic events.

Working With Greg, and My First Book Sale

THE COUNTDOWN TO NOVEMBER'S SKUSA SUPERNATS LASTED an eternity. So much had happened since Tom Kutscher broke the news at the I-55 podium ceremony in June. It felt as if it were three lifetimes ago. Also, I started to struggle working with Greg as my ability to communicate the challenges of the autism spectrum started to grow.

As difficult a time as I was having, Greg had it beat. He was under immense stress. Actually, immense stress doesn't begin to describe how bad a time he was going through. A year prior, two people joined his company as investors, which seemed like a godsend as the 2008 financial crisis hit and people scaled back their racing budgets. They had a grand plan for karting in the St. Louis area, including building a full-fledged CIK-FIA international grade track. Greg wanted me to run the competition side of the property. I was hesitant; I'd had so many things fall apart. My feeling was, I'd believe it when I saw it. It got close—there were blueprints, a zoning permit hearing—but as time went on, there were cracks showing in the framework.

Eventually, all sorts of charges were filed on these investors, and their story ended up on CNBC's *American Greed* series, with an image of Greg's go karts. As the arm of justice swooped in, we lost our great office space in Wentzville, and moved to Illinois.

Over the years, and the thousands of miles I'd ridden with Greg, I had explained autism the best I could at that time, but my inability to communicate on the fly remained a hindrance. Once, coming home from a race in Iowa, we stopped for the night in an RV park. We started discussing something he had asked me to do, and it turned out that there had been a miscommunication; I thought I had done what he'd asked, but I had not. Later that same week, he asked me to bring some items from the shop to the office, but once I got out to the shop, I'd forgotten what the items were. I went back into the office to ask exactly what he wanted, and once I was in the shop, you guessed it, I'd again forgotten what items to bring. Why didn't I just write them down? I don't know. After the third time, I just grabbed some random items and hoped for the best. It was a frustrating experience for both Greg and me.

It can be difficult for all parties when Asperger's is involved. When Greg saw me at the track, flags in hand, he was looking at a self-assured, soaring individual; he once told me that I "oozed confidence" when working as an official. Yet in the office, I was quiet, meek, and prone to errors. He knew the office wasn't my area of expertise, but in a work environment it's easy for the lines to blur between what a person is good at and what a person is not good at. I'd get frustrated myself as to why I could do certain difficult things with ease, and yet struggle with mundane, everyday tasks. This might be the most difficult thing for "normal" society to understand about people on the autism spectrum.

With that issue, and the trouble with his investors, Greg and I decided to terminate our employment arrangement; I would continue my racing duties, and be on call after races to handle bookkeeping. This was fine for me, except that it created an income problem, which didn't seem as bad as the stress the job had been creating. Besides, I didn't want to jeopardize my friendship with Greg.

At the end of September, we headed to Odessa, Missouri, for a SKUSA CSC race at I-70 Speedway. This was the wildest track I'd ever flagged at, incorporating the 30-degree banking of its famed oval track. We had to install multiple chicanes to cut the speeds. There was something extremely *retro* about this track that I appreciated. The fact that my "flagstand" was me standing on the narrow concrete wall made things interesting.

But maybe the most memorable thing about that I-70 weekend was that I sold my first batch of books. A week earlier, I had received my first shipment of *Finding Kansas*. My years of writing had turned into a real book, and my story could now be read by anyone. I sold about 30 books, which equated to $700. I couldn't believe it. More amazing still was the fact that those folks who bought copies wanted me to sign them. It was humbling, it was exciting, and I couldn't believe that all those late nights writing my thoughts, feelings, and hopes had turned into something tangible. It was also gratifying when I started getting messages from people who bought the book and said they loved it.

It was an encouraging end to the Midwest race season for me. Now my eyes were set on Las Vegas. I told Greg that I expected the SuperNats job to be easy, because I would only be flagging. He said, "Are you serious, you think it'll be easy?"

I said, "Of course. All I've got to do is wave the flag when they tell me to. How hard could it be?"

Famous last words …

SKUSA SuperNationals XII: My Arrival on the International Scene

AS NOVEMBER APPROACHED, I EMAILED TOM KUTSCHER'S wife, Patti, and asked if I should arrange my own travel to Las Vegas. I was shocked when she said that they'd buy me an airline ticket. Not only was I going to be paid to flag this major event, something I'd have paid *them* to do, but they were also going to pay for my flight and hotel. This was straight out of a dream.

That year's SKUSA SuperNationals took place at the Rio All-Suite Hotel & Casino, which meant we could walk to the track from our room. It was a surreal experience, strolling over to the pit area on the day before the race. I had to quietly take back what I told Greg Yocom about this being "easy" when I saw hundreds of team trailers in the parking lot, and the extremely technical track. Furthermore, I didn't know anyone on the staff. I was an outsider who took the place of someone who was still on staff, so I might have to also play the social game.

If my nerves weren't already high enough, the night before the start of the event we had an all-staff meeting. Many people spoke, among them long-time karting announcer Rob Howden, who reminded us that "the eyes of the karting world are on this event. Everything you do will be watched and critiqued." Goodness.

After the meeting, Tom Kutscher introduced me to Jim Holloway, vice president of Mothers Polish, and mentioned that I had a book coming out about the autism spectrum. This piqued Jim's interest, and he began asking a bunch of questions about the challenges faced by people on the spectrum. It felt natural interacting in this way and it was only later that I could look back on our exchange and say that I might have been giving my first presentation on this matter. As important as it was for me to work this event, this conversation with Jim Holloway helped pave the way for what was to come.

But first, I had to survive my rookie SuperNats.

It's hard to appreciate the shock to the system that comes with the first green flag, when 40 karts take to the track for practice. The most karts I'd ever had on a track I flagged was about 24, so this was an eye-opener. I was also tasked with making sure the track was clear after each session and releasing the grid for the next session via radio. Again, this was a night-and-day change from the smaller regional stuff I'd done. And staff? On the radio were at least a dozen corner workers, three different race directors, plus officials handling scoring, the grid, the scales, and more. I was thrown into the fire, and I maintained my composure and survived the morning session.

Rob Howden's words kept echoing in my head. I thought about how much style I should put into my flagging. No, I wasn't there to put on a flagman's clinic; the important part of the job is communicating with the drivers via the flags. At the same time, it was my style that got me there. I do know that I flagged with too much urgency in practice. Later, I was exhausted.

That first night, the former flagger and his friend talked to me. The conversation started out nicely enough, but then the friend said, "The way you clear the track and the way you talk are not appreciated. You should be quiet." This was sudden, it was loud enough for others to hear, and I didn't know how to react. The lead race director had no issues with the job I did, so to have a co-worker criticize me like that was a shock to the system. I didn't react for fear of *over-reacting*, so I did nothing. I maintained my composure.

The next morning, a woman from Rock Island, Illinois, a corner worker, approached me and said, "Don't listen to them, Aaron. You're doing fantastic, and we all know it. Keep it up!" It's amazing how one bit of encouragement can turn the tide. I wish I'd heard that the night before; I struggled to sleep, worried that this man's words might lead to the end of my job. As you've probably picked up by now, we on the autism spectrum can be catastrophic thinkers.

The SuperNationals were four days long, and day two featured qualifying and the first round of heat races. By now, I *knew* that my guess about this being easy couldn't have been more wrong. The drivers were overly aggressive and didn't respect each other or the confines of the track. We had incident after incident, and the red flag was needed far too often. It was a true test of my ability to stay calm.

The next day proved to be a learning experience on many fronts. Ideally, the experience you gain at previous jobs will set you up with the knowledge you'll need for your dream job, because there would be nothing worse than to get your dream job and discover that you don't have the full skill set. Day three at the SuperNats would teach me two things.

During the afternoon, there was a multi-kart crash in the chicane. In every race I'd ever worked, I had the authority to throw a red flag if I thought one was needed. Here, that was up to the race director. During this crash and the ensuing cleanup, a corner worker in that turn started waving a red flag. There was a lot of radio chatter, and it was difficult to know if an official red had been called. But seeing his red flag, I picked up mine and gave it a couple of twirls. Just then, the corner worker who'd been waving his red flag withdrew it. What was going on? An inadvertent red could easily bring grief to competitors and to the staff and would be a bad thing to be blamed for. Somehow, no drivers saw the red flags and the race proceeded with no one disadvantaged. After that, I made sure to wait until hearing from the sole person in charge.

The official red flags kept coming, pushing the program deeper into the night. Floodlights were on hand and racing at night was sensory bliss, from the smoke rolling off the grid to the showers of sparks when karts bottomed out.

The junior class was up for their second heat, and as the previous race finished, I heard the familiar thud of a kart hitting a Tecpro barrier close to me. Once you've heard that sound, you'll recognize it every time. But I looked around and saw nothing, no karts spun around or crashed.

I took my place, green flag in hand, and as the field reached the next-to-last corner, I saw what had made the noise: a kart had indeed hit a section of Tecpro, which itself pushed against a highway barrier and moved it slightly. Now the blunt end of that barrier was sticking out into the racing line at the apex of turn one; barely, yes, but it was sticking out. I thought about radioing the race director or waving off the start, but this was so minor I was sure I'd be chastised for the delay. So, I waved the green, and shortly thereafter I was running for my life.

The fourth-place starter clipped the end of that barrier, which took the left-rear wheel clean off his kart with the precision of a vegetable slicer. He spun in front of 36 other karts, and the ensuing pile up was one sickening impact after another. The wall I was running away from kept getting slammed into, and it almost clipped me. I looked over my shoulder and saw one kart drive up and over another kart and its driver.

Once the last kart had joined in the crash, I jumped over the wall to assist. I was sure that there had to be drivers hurt, perhaps seriously. I went first to the driver who'd just been run over; he had a tire mark on the face shield of his helmet. I asked if he was okay, and his reaction was, "Can my dad fix my kart?"

Okay kid, you're fine.

Then one of Greg Yocom's drivers came up and asked, "Can I fix my bumper?" It was becoming clear that, somehow, there were no injuries, and each kid's only concern was to get back in the race. The ensuing debate on whether the rules allowed repairs was one I was happy not to be a part of. But the valuable lesson, for me, concerned the *cause* of the wreck, and the lesson was this: If you see something, say something. I doubt we'd have waved off the start to push the wall back a couple of inches, but it might have saved some karts had everyone been aware of the situation before the field was coming to the green.

Super Sunday came, and again I learned a huge lesson. Shortly into the junior race, there was a red flag. Drivers swarmed the race director asking if there would be a complete restart, or a restart with one lap complete; each situation meant a slightly different running order. The race director called for a complete restart, and several drivers started screaming at him. In my view, the field had been on its second lap, so surely one lap had been completed. I asked the race director, "Complete restart? How does that work?" He turned from the drivers, pointed a finger at me, and yelled, "F***, Aaron! We're supposed to be on the same team!"

Same team? I hadn't meant my questioning of his call as a criticism. I simply wanted him to be right, so I needed to understand his thinking on this. But the way I went about this, appearing to disagree with him in front of those angry competitors, was not a good look.

The race director later apologized for his outburst, and I apologized as well.

With the final races on tap, I started fearing the end. The

catastrophic thinker in me felt like this was it; I'd never get to do this again. Dan Wheldon and Jamie McMurray raced in that year's SuperNationals, and I worried that I'd never again work a race with names as big as theirs. And that fear brought out some flair: I started stepping over the Tecpro barrier to display my double checkered flags. No one yelled at me for it, and it felt much more natural for me than flagging from behind a wall.

Soon enough, the event was over. I survived, although I now experienced a level of exhaustion I'd never known. The next night's flight home was the loneliest of my life. There was a joy in being tested in every aspect of physical and mental wherewithal, on that big a stage. It felt like a drug, and it seemed to be an addictive drug. For the first time in my life, I found something as enjoyable as being in the driver's seat. And, hell, this was harder!

The plane touched down in Saint Louis, and my dad picked me up. I sat in silence, holding back the kind of tears you get after you've experienced heaven.

2009: A New Purpose

ALL THE QUESTIONS I HAD ABOUT WHAT I WAS GOING TO DO with my life came to a head and were answered in 2009. In life, you can be on a journey whose destination you don't know, but after you arrive, you'll see how everything put you on the path you needed to be on. That's what happened in 2009.

I had my first book signing at a Barnes & Noble in St. Louis. A family I met there—the first family I ever met as an author—had a horror story about their son and their inability to get an autism diagnosis for him. According to these people, the school district refused to give a diagnosis for two reasons: "One, he can talk; two he gets good grades, so even if he has autism, which he doesn't, he'll outgrow it by age 16." I was flabbergasted at such a ridiculous claim.

At that same book signing, a man was hovering around my table with a puzzled look. He watched as I engaged with parents and individuals on the spectrum. During a lull, he came up and said, "I don't believe you're on the autism spectrum." Come again? I froze, tried to speak, but hesitated. He said, "Yes, how are you doing this? A person on the spectrum can't do this."

Once I had the composure to respond, I mentioned what I called my "Alias concept," which says that I can do this sort of thing when I have a role to play. I could have used the example of myself as a race director holding a drivers' meeting, but to fit this setting I said that at the moment I was not the everyday, ordinary Aaron Likens, but rather "Aaron the author guy who seems to know what he's talking about." This opened up a dialogue, and the man mentioned that he was a professor at nearby Lindenwood University and perhaps we should stay in touch.

From that book signing came another, this one at a non-profit in St. Louis which at the time was called Judevine Center for Autism. At that second signing, I met a man who would soon change my life, Ron Ekstrand, who worked with the Judevine Center and also with Easterseals. Ron said that he'd read my book and was captivated by the way I turned long clinical explanations into easy-to-explain metaphors. He asked if I'd be willing to go through their parent-training program and give feedback on how they might incorporate my concepts into their curriculum. I had held several job titles, but never "consultant," so I was happy to say yes.

Participating in that program, I felt that for the first time in my life I was getting accurate information on autism. Before that, I had subscribed mostly to the info I found on that awful non-medical website in the week after my diagnosis in 2003. Going through the Judevine Center's multi-week program, and learning that I could only be defined by my diagnosis if *I* allowed it, was monumental.

It was also during that program that I looked on as a 5-year-old girl spoke for the first time—*said her very first word!*—with her mother there in the room. It was impossible not to be impacted by seeing this girl make that step and witnessing her mother's tearful reaction.

The Indianapolis 500 that year proved to be an emotional one. My dad had another commitment on the day of the race, so for the first time I'd be going to the 500 by myself.

I've mentioned that I get emotional during the pre-race ceremonies at Indy, but this year that feeling was even more intense. Perhaps it was because I was taking in those moments—the playing of "Taps," the National Anthem, and "Back Home Again in Indiana"—alone for the very first time. You look around the Speedway and realize that in the hundreds of thousands of people sharing the same emotions, there are fathers and sons, and grandfathers with their sons and grandsons, and maybe one of those grandsons is attending his *first* 500. Sometime in the future, there will come a day when those families come to the track on race day with one family member missing. While my dad is still alive, that race in 2009 gave me the sense of what it might be like someday without him; it was because of him that my interest in the Indianapolis 500 got started in the first place, and we have shared so many great moments at the race. He was not beside me that day in 2009, but it felt as if he was beside me during the pre-race ceremonies. I'm sure it will always feel that way.

The next day, I headed east with a couple of items on my agenda. First, I visited an aunt in Washington, D.C., and together we went to the next weekend's NASCAR Cup race in Dover, Delaware. That might not have been the greatest choice of places to take her, because my aunt's favorite sport is tennis, and there's a big difference between Wimbledon and the Dover International Speedway. It probably didn't help that the race was not very exciting; Jimmie Johnson dominated, leading 298 of the 400 laps. But my boredom gave me some time to reflect on the previous few months of my life, with the Judevine training program I'd been part of, my own discoveries about autism, and the book signings that allowed me to hear stories from families with loved ones on the autism spectrum. These reflections drove home the fact that there was something solid to my work. Jimmie Johnson won yet another NASCAR race that day, and I'm sure he brought a lot of happiness to those on his team, but I can't imagine that it matched the happiness of seeing a 5-year-old say her first words.

I felt as if I was finding my purpose.

The main point of my trip to the East Coast was to go to New York City and meet the researcher with whom my dad had corresponded in 2006, sending her some of my early writings. She had offered words of encouragement back then, and she ended up writing an endorsement for *Finding Kansas*, a book that might not have existed without encouraging words from her and only a few others.

She was working at the headquarters of Autism Speaks, so the meeting was at their office in the city. Driving into and through Manhattan was intimidating; I had butterflies, much like I had in my first race. And the visit, too, was a source of intimidation. This researcher was a doctor, an expert in her field, and I was, well, just an Aspie from St. Louis. Why did I deserve this type of meeting?

Meeting her was another gate I passed through in the progression of my life. She mentioned how much she learned from my book, and how I helped shape her thoughts about the hidden emotions a person on the spectrum may have. In her office that day, she asked me a life-changing question: "Aaron, now that you have a book, do you still want to race?"

I smiled and thought back to that parent-training program, and I said, "Yes, I still want to race, but it's a *new* race now. I didn't know it for most of my life, but there is so much hope for those on the autism spectrum … but only if society is aware of its existence.

"Parents out there are being told that their kid will simply 'outgrow' autism, but the spectrum is like wet cement: We've got to work with it while it's wet, before it sets and is like stone. So, I still want to race, but the race is to spread as much understanding as possible."

With that spoken paragraph, I realized that I finally wanted something more than to stand in victory lane after the Indianapolis 500 with a wreath around my neck, taking the traditional sip of milk, hearing the roar of the crowd. Instead, I wanted to have a positive impact on families, and use the things I'd learned and the concepts I had to … *to make a difference.*

The drive back to St. Louis was much longer than the mileage indicated because much of it was spent in deep thought. For the second time in my life, I was in a position of having talent and ambition with no way to showcase it. But this time, instead of lacking a race car, I had no platform, no stage, to help spread the understanding I now had.

Triumph Amid Defeat

A COUPLE OF WEEKS LATER, I TOOK PART IN A CONFERENCE in downtown St. Louis where I'd have books for sale. My confidence was soaring; when your desire has concrete results, in my case a published book, well, surely glory comes easily, right? I was on my way to becoming a *name*, and this conference would be the next lap towards reaching the heights I knew I was headed for, simply because I wanted it.

The morning of the conference, as my dad and I drove downtown, there wasn't an inch of doubt in my mind as to what was going to happen. I hadn't yet heard from other authors about the difficulties of selling books if the setting isn't perfect, for whatever reason. This isn't to deter you if you want to be an author. Just don't go into a conference *expecting* results.

My book was nicely displayed, but I can recall person after person looking at me, then looking at the book, and moving on while I stood there awkwardly. Each snub hurt me. What was going on? Was this journey all for naught? Already I'd forgotten my sales at prior signings.

My dad tried to help, but there was no change in the demeanor of the attendees. Maybe if I'd been a cardboard cutout, I'd have stoked more conversations. After three hours, there had been not a single conversation and not a single book sale. It was an utter strikeout. My dreams of book sales and whatever passion I'd conveyed to the doctor in New York were dying.

The next week was torture. Was I destined to discover that I could be good at things, but never be able to fully enjoy them? Why have skills if you couldn't use them? My skill set is narrow, but when I'm good at something, I can excel. The thought of enduring another decade spent trying to break into another profession wasn't something I smiled about.

A week after the book signing, my dad told me that we'd be dropping in on that professor from Lindenwood University and his master's-level teaching course. I couldn't fathom why I'd have any interest in "dropping in" on such a thing. He also told me to wear a nice shirt, which was perplexing.

When that night arrived, I put on nice pants and a nice shirt, and headed up to Lindenwood University in St. Charles. I still wasn't sure why we were going. Halfway there, my dad said, "So, that professor read your book, and he's using it in his class." Wow! To know that people I'd never met were reading about my journey through Asperger's was great.

"And by the way," said my dad, "the professor asked if you'd talk about your book. I made a PowerPoint presentation you can look at before you begin."

Say again? Wait, please don't! I couldn't possibly give a presentation about myself.

I looked out the window, wanting to jump out and run. Panic was creeping in, and this was looking like a panic attack to the core. Standing in front of others seemed like an impossible task. Yes, I had conducted many drivers' meetings, but that was different. At the race track, I wasn't talking about myself, about my hopes, dreams, and challenges. My book was meant to be a one-way medium, to be enjoyed by the reader without me present.

At Lindenwood, I looked across the campus and jokingly asked my dad, "Can I run *that* way? I bet I'd set a new record." He didn't see the humor, and said, "You're doing this." I wasn't given an option.

I reviewed my dad's PowerPoint presentation, and its flow was perfect, addressing all the main concepts in my book. All I had to do for the students was connect the dots and tell my story. Well, who better to tell my story than me? I knew the source material quite well.

The professor told the audience his story of meeting me, and how he didn't understand how a person with Asperger's could be "normal" in one setting and not in another. He said that in reading my book, he was impressed with my ability to put into language anyone could understand the challenges and the concepts I used for facing those challenges.

Then, after an intro, it was my turn. I could feel each drop of blood in my body flowing. The pulse in my neck was beating like a drum, my toes were numb, and I was not breathing properly. You want to talk about stage fright? This was the epitome of it. I was not cut out for this, and I was sure it was going to end like the book signing had: in abject failure.

But as I introduced myself, somehow my words started to … *flow*. It was as if I were writing, one sentence after another, on a computer screen. I suppose it was something like driving a race car, in that I was not *overthinking* anything. I had never before given a presentation, yet it felt as if I were speaking from a script that I'd read and rehearsed a thousand times. Well, why not? This script was *my life*.

I was a hit. The professor had to cut off the subsequent Q&A segment of the program, because too many students had questions. And I was *loving* it!

Later, the professor said, "Aaron, you have a future in this, and I hope I'm around to see it."

In the car, my dad revealed that he'd known for over a week about the professor's plan for this night. He didn't want to tell me, because he knew I'd panic and not do it, so he put me in a situation where I had no choice. He said, "Aaron, in your book you wrote, 'In situations where it's sink or swim, I always swim.' So, I made this a situation where you had to swim."

He was right. I'm not suggesting that this tactic would work for others, but for me, that was the only way to do it. In one night, I proved to myself that I had the ability to make public presentations. I'd been worrying that I'd never find a platform to spread the things I'd learned, and now I had one.

The Big Time

OCTOBER AND NOVEMBER OF 2009 WERE THE LAST STAGES of the rollercoaster I'd been on. In science terms, potential energy was turning into kinetic energy in both my professions. It started with a presentation booked with help from Ron Ekstrand and a grandmother who'd been part of the parent-training program I went through. This grandmother was a member of the Missouri National Educators Association, and it was her suggestion that I participate in a conference that drew 500 teachers. She'd never seen me present, but she loved the book, and now that I knew I had the ability to do this, I said yes. I'd also help work a booth with Matt Schafer, Judevine's new community-education specialist.

I knew nothing about the services provided, and I did not know Matt, but on my first day at this conference he was very open about how much he learned from my book, and that he hoped we'd make a good team. He was right about that. I wish I could say that I went in and threw a perfect game, but it was the conversations set up by Matt that gave me confidence. These teachers knew far more than I, and yet they seemed to hang on every word and story I said. At times, our booth had so many people that we were encroaching on the booths beside us, and we got some nasty looks from those on either side of us.

After a couple of days, it was my turn to speak in the ballroom. Attendees had told me that after speaking to me in person, they switched their schedules to attend my presentation instead of the one they'd originally selected. Still, I was worried no one would show up, and I had a partially revamped PowerPoint that I hadn't reviewed because, well, I was nervous again. A fear of public speaking isn't something you get over just because you impressed 15 or so college students.

I didn't go near or enter the ballroom until three minutes before my scheduled start time. I had prepared myself for a strikeout like the one I'd had at that book signing, but as I neared the room, I saw a line to get in. And when I walked through the doors, it was clear that the room was on its way to filling to its absolute capacity; once those people in the hall got in, the place would be packed. There was a buzz in the air as folks awaited the event.

As I walked towards the front of the room, I felt a strange hush. Someone said that word had gotten around that there was a new speaker, that some of the people I'd spoken with at the booth had passed word to their friends, and that my event had become the must-see presentation of the conference. The grandmother who'd arranged all of this introduced me and remarked that she couldn't recall a presentation as highly anticipated as this one.

Thanks, I thought. As if I wasn't nervous enough.

This was a full-length presentation, and along the way I lost all sense of time. As it came to the end, I thought I'd done a horrible job. But as I was closing out by thanking them all for attending, my words were lost in the noise. Everyone stood, and there was a chorus of applause. I looked to my left, then my right, hoping to find someone who would tell me what to do next. But this roar of applause just kept coming.

A bit lost, I walked awkwardly out of the room and went back to the booth where Matt asked, "How'd it go?" I said that I didn't know, and that was an honest answer. But then people who'd seen the presentation started showing up at the booth to buy my book and ask me questions. Matt said, "Aaron, it would appear that your presentation was a major hit."

Several weeks later, I was off to Las Vegas to flag my second SKUSA SuperNationals. There was an extra buzz around this year's edition because the entries included seven-time Formula 1 World Champion Michael Schumacher. Michael had stepped away from Formula 1 after the 2006 season, but there had recently been rumors that he would make a 2010 comeback, which he announced a month after the SuperNats. The media attention around Schumacher's appearance was incredible.

I was asked to speak at the drivers' meeting, discussing flagging procedures. I'll never forget one of the race directors, Terry Bybee, introducing me with the words, "Everyone listen up! This is Aaron, and I assure you, you'll see him flag at Indianapolis one day."

Every SuperNats is a big deal, but Schumacher's presence magnified everything. When I flagged the class he was in, I actually had to work around media personnel who congregated at the start/finish line. Each time he took to the track, there was no room to spectate; every spot was taken, in no small part by the racers and teams competing in other classes.

On track, Schumacher had an atrocious week, with mechanical breakdowns in practice and qualifying. Each time he slowed to a stop, it was like every worker on duty wanted to help him; there'd be six people around the kart when two could have done the job. The nice thing was, Michael never accepted the help. He may have been one of the highest-paid sports stars in history, but in Las Vegas he tried hard to be just another kart racer who deserved no special attention. On the final day, he made it a point to shake the hands of all the workers.

For me, the 2009 SuperNats was an opposite experience from the '08 version. The red flag stayed in its place, instead of flying every other session. I really enjoyed that.

While I was in Vegas, and without knowing about it, my dad made a phone call to the Indianapolis Motor Speedway Museum to speak with Donald Davidson, the popular track historian. Donald was one of the few non-500-winners I asked to sign the checkered flag given to me by Duane Sweeney.

My dad had phoned Donald to ask a simple question: "If someone wanted to one day have a chance at flagging the Indianapolis 500, how should they go about it?"

Donald's suggestion was that it would be smart to work through the United Stated Auto Club, because USAC had long been a stepping stone not only for starters but for race officials in general. He added that paying dues at the local short tracks, where officials might be paid little if they were paid at all, might also be helpful.

Each year, my dad and I had been spending Thanksgiving with my aunt in Washington, D.C., which meant that we'd be heading east the day I got home from Las Vegas. This time, the trip would take just a little bit longer, because on the way there I'd be having a meeting with USAC's senior vice president of racing operations, Jason Smith, at the sanctioning body's office in Indianapolis.

I can only guess how many people ask USAC and its officials, "Hey, how does one get into flagging?" But, having just worked the SKUSA SuperNationals with Michael Schumacher in the field gave me an extra talking point, and Jason and I did talk about that.

He asked me how long I'd been starting races, and I said, "Since 1995."

"Goodness," said Jason, "you have more years of experience than *most* of my flaggers!"

He added, "What are you doing this week? I need someone for Turkey Night." He meant the Turkey Night Grand Prix, one of the nation's most prestigious Midget races, which in that period ran at California's Irwindale Speedway. I gave Jason sort of a flaky answer because I was caught off guard but also because I didn't want to screw up our Thanksgiving tradition.

Not only that, but I also wasn't sure that being thrown straight into an event like Turkey Night would be the best course of action.

I thought the meeting went well, and at the end Jason asked me if I knew anything about Quarter Midgets. I did not, but he mentioned that USAC had started a national series for those cars and that they'd been busy forming a staff. He said that maybe he'd get me in touch with them at some point in time. He also suggested that I "shadow" his USAC staffers at a couple of races to get a feel for things, and mentioned that the Indiana events in May, all running in the buildup to the Indianapolis 500, would be a great time to do that.

The USAC office is just across 16th Street from the Indianapolis Motor Speedway, and as we left the meeting it seemed to me like things were looking up. And so was I; yes, I was looking at the huge Speedway grandstands, wondering if one day, instead of sitting in a reserved seat, I might be working there on race day.

I felt as if my hopes and dreams had a chance.

Being Given a Chance to Swing for the Fences

THE RESPONSE I'D GOTTEN FROM MY PRESENTATION FOR THE Missouri National Educators Association and Matt's praise for the work we'd done together at the conference did not go unnoticed by the Judevine Center for Autism, known today as TouchPoint Autism Services. As 2009 ended, I had a job interview with Ron Ekstrand, who said during the interview that he wasn't sure what my job would even look like. He told me that a vice president in the organization had agreed to do some POST training—Peace Officer Standards and Training—for the St. Louis County Police Academy, as part of the continuing education officers need when interacting with the public. This VP hadn't realized that it involved 35 sessions at random intervals in the first five months of 2010. It might be two days a week, or one day, or four. Ron asked if I'd be willing to work part-time on these sessions. I said yes, then wondered if I had anything to offer these officers.

I was supplied with a PowerPoint, but I barely glanced at it before my first presentation. It occurs to me now that maybe this goes back to my racing days; I hated practice and glancing at this PowerPoint seemed like practice. I'd rather just be thrown into the fire!

Before my first presentation, I drove to the academy shaking with stage fright. As usual, I thought my presentation to these police officers was rocky. There was a section where I wanted to illustrate the point that people on the autism spectrum may not understand social situations, and I told the story about sending a breakup text message to my girlfriend on Christmas. The officers responded with a rumble of laughter. I thought, "Why are they laughing? This isn't funny." When I added, "And I broke up just to see if she still liked me," there was another eruption of laughs. Some other situations I mentioned later brought more chuckling. I was sure that I had bombed. Why else would they laugh?

I left quickly, so I missed a chance to speak with Sgt. Barry Armfield, who was the head of the St. Louis Police Department's Crisis Intervention Team. The sergeant liked my presentation so much that he wanted me to repeat it to all the CIT classes in the area. Once again, I'd been a hit without realizing it.

With each police presentation, I worked on my timing. Since the laughter was usually at the same place, I added some pauses. It actually began to feel natural, easy, and I loved it. There were officers who had kids on the spectrum and said that I'd brought them some hope—which to me was hard to grasp because I had so often been without hope myself. A year earlier, I had almost no prospects, and now I was training police officers on how to handle themselves and others in what could be life-or-death situations. While I enjoyed bringing some energy and laughter, it wasn't lost on me how serious this work was.

A month or so into all of this, there was another meeting with Ron Ekstrand. He told me that his offer of a part-time job was off the table; instead, he proposed that I come to work full time, even though he still didn't know exactly what my job would be. I'd never had a full-time job in my life. Ron said that it might take us a while to get rolling, but if I had the patience, he thought we would change the world … or at least Missouri.

How could I say no? I told Ron about my commitments to the new SKUSA Pro Tour and the SuperNationals, and that I was hoping to work some USAC events. He told me not to worry, because my racing duties would be part of our story.

Looking back on this, Ron's moves here were pivotal to both my presenting and racing careers. He saw the potential I had, when I saw none. So many of the stories of success I tell have a Ron or a Greg in them, because I am not self-made. So often in life, forward moves are aided by "who you know," so it's important to meet and speak with the right people when you can. Without those people, many of us fall into a familiar trap: We know that we'd be able to handle a certain job, but we won't ever get that chance. I will forever be grateful for the doors Ron Ekstrand opened for me, doors that opened onto the path to my full potential.

— Establishing a Voice at Home and Away —

I TOOK A SMALL DETOUR IN FEBRUARY OF 2010, AND WENT to Vancouver for the Winter Olympics. When I landed back in St. Louis, I was a full-time employee ... and it felt great.

Well, at least it did for a little while. Four hours after my return, I had to make a presentation at the police academy, and it had a much different feel from the others I'd given. When I arrived at the academy to speak, the opening slide of my PowerPoint presentation was on the screen. A high-ranking officer was in the second row; in other words, not too far from my position. He saw what was on the screen, looked around, and said, "Hey guys, get a load of this! Autism? What a bunch of spoiled children!"

I didn't know how to react. Even though I'd had some great, well-received presentations, I was still a rookie, unsure of how I came across. And here was this officer, undermining me.

As I went along, this same officer gave me a disapproving shake of his head each time I made a point. I was jet-lagged, and exhausted from being awake for well over 24 hours. The beauty of the closing ceremonies at the Olympics, with its amazing fireworks display over BC Place, was now replaced by this disrespectful police officer. Normally, this same program would take 50 minutes, but on this day it lasted just 35.

I've now given over 1,000 presentations, and this was the only time my message was mocked. But that day, perhaps because I was still somewhat new to this, I allowed doubt to creep into my head. Was I a bad presenter? Today I'd know how to handle this situation, but I did not yet have the confidence to go toe-to-toe with this man. The next day I spoke about it with Matt, and he gave me a pep talk, warning me about the dark hearts that wouldn't be receptive to a message like mine. He said that I should instead focus on those I *was* reaching.

Matt then told me about a tour he and I were going to make, visiting doctors' offices in the St. Louis area to let them know that we were a resource they could rely on. As part of these visits, the pediatricians and nurses could pick my brain on anything autism-related. We called these "lunch-and-learn" sessions, with us providing lunch for those in the office.

I felt like I was mastering the art of talking to an audience solo, so being half of a two-person team did not come naturally to me. But Matt helped me so much when we did these lunch-and learn sessions, providing seamless tosses to me that allowed me to answer and engage without much effort. It was eerie how great he was at being the wingman; he'd begin talking and then step aside to allow me to shine. We were like Ed McMahon and Johnny Carson. I think we really made a difference that allowed the staffs at these offices to better understand and even diagnose autism. Matt's grace and lack of ego helped build my confidence, and this even helped make my police presentations better.

A month into my full-time job, I had my first SKUSA Pro Tour race at Sonoma Raceway in California. This was a treat for me, but I still worried about how it would impact my full-time job. I was assured that as long as I blogged about it, it was considered work, and thus began my pattern of blogging at airports, in this case Oakland International.

That first Pro Tour weekend was memorable, because I was able to perform what I called my "playing in traffic" start, something I'd first done at the SuperNationals. On rolling starts I'd be standing almost in the center of the track, and as the field crept toward me I'd fly the green flag high and then run off the track. Was it an adrenaline rush? Yes, so much so that I'm writing this with a giant smile on my face. Maybe this was what a matador feels as a bull rushes by. That kind of start required a lot of focus; it's like everything in the world has ceased to exist except me, my green flag, and that field of karts.

Were these starts dangerous? Well, yes. When my mom saw a photo from the SuperNats, her instructions were, "Quit it!"

She may have had a point. My mom was listening to
the Sonoma broadcast on ekartingnews.com when, on the
opening green flag for a junior-class feature, the driver starting fourth tried to overtake both front-row karts, creating a
three-wide situation. But two of the karts touched and shot
straight in my direction. I was already running away from
the track, but here they came, right at me. My only option
was to jump. The problem with jumping is that you only
get one chance to get it right; once you're in the air, you are
no longer in control. So my timing had to be perfect, or the
injuries might be extensive. Three, two, one … *JUMP.*

It was a good jump, because I avoided being badly hurt.
But I still ended up on the ground, unable to breathe. My
mom heard the announcer Rob Howden's call: "There's
contact at the start, two karts spinning and … Oh! They've
clipped starter Aaron Likens, who is down."

My legs were okay, my arms were okay. But while it
looked like I had been struck, I had not. I just landed badly
and speared myself with one of the flags, which knocked
the wind out of me. I felt my phone vibrating in my pocket,
which turned out to be mom texting to see if I was okay. As
other officials hovered over me, I heard a voice on the radio
ask, "Do we need to go red?" I wasn't going to be the cause
of a red flag, so I hopped up, hobbled back to the finish line
and spent the rest of that heat trying to catch my breath.

Another memory from that weekend is an argument my
black flag caused with Colton Herta and his dad, Bryan. The
black-flag procedure was as follows: A rolled-up flag pointed
at a driver is just a warning, but if a black is being waved
ferociously, it means that we want you in the pits right now.
After I pointed a warning flag at Colton, he pulled into the
pits and lost many positions. When they were informed
that he'd only received a warning flag and didn't need to
pit, Bryan and Colton said that I had waved the flag, and I
maintained that I hadn't. But life went on, and Colton has

done okay for himself since; he's one of the top drivers in IndyCar.

The Monday after the race, I did my first blog post from the airport. It dealt with the weekend's races, the joys of traveling, the ways autism *helps* me at the track, and something my mom had told me in another text: "Aaron, didn't I tell you not to play in traffic?"

Yes, she had. But I'd been playing in traffic since I found that rock in front of my house and turned it into a flagstand when I was just a boy. I had no intentions of stopping now.

Thursday, Friday, and Saturday Night Thunder

IN THE WEEK LEADING UP TO THE 2010 INDIANAPOLIS 500, I had my first assignments from USAC, working for three straight nights as assistant starter for all of the organization's national divisions: Sprint Cars at the Terre Haute Action Track on Thursday, the Hoosier Hundred for Silver Crown cars at the Indiana State Fairgrounds on Friday, and the "Night Before the 500" Midget classic at Indianapolis Raceway Park on Saturday. Growing up, watching USAC races in the "Thunder" events on ESPN was a weekly habit for me.

Heading into Terre Haute, I had no instructions other than "be there at 5:00 p.m." I didn't know what I'd be doing, or with whom I'd be working. The program got off to a strange start; it was almost a man-made rainout. Dirt tracks need water, but this one had been *over*-watered. Parts of the track were basically flooded. I hadn't been given a radio yet, so I watched from the infield and wondered if the track would ever be ready. In time, with help from a lot of cars, trucks, and track vehicles making laps, the track was finally in shape for racing.

The Terre Haute flagstand is barely big enough for one person, so I was stationed inside the first turn with a directive to "observe and listen to radio protocols." As the heat races began, you couldn't have wiped the smile off my face. The ground shook from the might of the engines, and the Sprint Cars entered the corner so sideways that it didn't seem real. I was overjoyed. As hard as I tried to just watch and listen, I'm sure the fan in me was showing.

The sun had long set when the feature race took to the track. I was amazed at how the USAC starter, Tom Hansing, commanded the radio when he spoke. He was clear, concise, and there was never any doubt as to what he expected. I worried that I'd never have that ability; I hadn't thought about that part of the job. This isn't to say I was unprofessional at SKUSA; it's just that things happen much faster on a half-mile dirt track, and Tom, who was also one of the IndyCar starters, was right on top of it all. If there was a flagman to learn from, it would certainly be Tom.

I had yet to speak on the radio as the green flag flew for the main event. By now, I was taking my directive very seriously; the fan in me had been muted, and I was an official, even if I was the assistant starter without a flag in the first-turn infield. I couldn't quite shake the image of playing baseball in third grade, when I was relegated to left field because no one ever hit the ball there. But at about the halfway mark of the race, I was glad to be where I was; my position as "observer" paid off when I watched one of the tail-end Sprint Cars "bicycle" onto its right-side wheels, and then flip up and over the barrier without touching it.

I heard nothing on the radio, and when I glanced toward Tom on the flagstand, I didn't see any movement. Could everyone but me have missed this? Well, it happened so fast that if I hadn't been looking right at that car when it took off, I'd have missed it myself. My instincts took over and I keyed the radio, shouting the same call I'd heard the regular officials use a few times earlier in the program.

"Red! Red! Red!"

The safety lights around the track went red, Tom Hansing waved his red flag, and for a few seconds there was confusion. There were no wrecked cars on the track, no visible emergency. The race director came on the radio and said, "Who the f*** called red? Why the f*** are we red?"

I'm sure it sounded like I had the meekest radio voice when I said, "Car over wall, turn one." Safety personnel were dispatched to that area, and people ran across the track to look over the barrier. A few moments later, sure enough, a helmeted figure appeared; the driver was okay, although the same could not be said for the pickup truck whose bed his Sprint Car landed in. I got a radio compliment for paying attention and for my quick call.

The next night, I was at the Indiana State Fairgrounds one-mile dirt track for the Hoosier Hundred. I had been to this race as a spectator for the past six years, but to go into the sign-in gate, pick up my pass as assistant starter, and walk around the infield pits was surreal. Again, I was a bit lost as to what to do or where to go. I hadn't been given any orders about whom to meet, or where to meet them. Racing jobs tend to be like this; every series has its regular officials who know the routine, and there aren't often newcomers. I stood around in full Aspie awkwardness.

Each minute seemed like an eternity. I may be competent and professional when I'm doing my job, but my discomfort in needing to ask for something, or someone, or for guidance, is an example of how difficult the "normal" can be for me. Thankfully, Tom Hansing recognized me from Terre Haute, and introduced himself. He didn't know me, but I felt as if I were meeting a legend; in just two days, he would be in the flagstand for the Indianapolis 500 as an assistant. I'm sure I stumbled upon every word as I introduced myself.

Along with the Silver Crown series, there was a UMP Modified race at the Fairgrounds, and Tom went across the track to flag their practice. I stayed in the infield, looking towards turn one and wondering if that would be my post here, too. About five minutes later I heard Tom on the radio, asking the race director for permission for me to cross the track and join him. I was in such a state of shock that I didn't hear the race director's response, but when I looked up at the flagstand I saw Tom looking in my direction and gesturing "come here." I looked around me and behind me, to be sure he wasn't signaling someone else. No, he wanted *me*. I crossed the track, stumbled a bit at the gate, and took my place beside Tom as he threw the green for practice.

Even after 15 years of flagging races, this new experience made me feel like I was starting all over. Speeds on the straightaway below me were over 120 miles per hour. To see the cars have wheelspin in a straight line, with the drivers feathering the throttle to get all the power to the track, was a perspective I had never seen. I didn't smile, I didn't frown; I was trying to soak in every second of this experience, because I was already fearing it might never happen again.

The practices came and went, and during intermission a person in a USAC polo shirt approached me. He introduced himself as James Spink, USAC's director of developmental series, who was overseeing the Quarter Midgets. James said that he'd heard from Jason Smith that I was interested in working with USAC. We talked a little bit about the Quarter Midgets; I didn't know much about those cars because my background had been in karts, but told him that I'd be up for something new. He seemed pleased and told me that if I was available, I could flag a race the following week. Well, I couldn't do that, because I would be in Kansas City to give some presentations; I had also signed on to do a race there with a karting club.

James said, "Well, we have our Battle at the Brickyard coming up in July. It's our largest Quarter Midget event. See you there." I wasn't offered a chance to say no; I was booked for a race at the Brickyard … also known as the Indianapolis Motor Speedway.

The Modified feature rolled out, and again I joined Tom in the stand. Ken Schrader dominated the 20-lap race, and after Schrader and a few other cars had taken the white flag, Tom did a no-look handoff and told me to wave it over the remainder of the field.

I put all of my style into waving that white flag. I felt as if every cell in my body was soaring and my soul had achieved perfect clarity. I had waved a flag at one of America's most historic auto-racing venues. I'd been awaiting this moment for almost my entire life. This doesn't in any way diminish the feelings I had for SKUSA, or for karting, but this was a one-mile track with full-sized race cars. I stepped back as Tom did a beautiful double-checkered wave over Schrader's winning car.

For the Silver Crown 100-mile race, I assisted Tom in keeping track of lapped traffic, and handing him the right flags at the right times, including the blue passing flag. It quickly became natural and effortless. Earlier, I'd been so clumsy just talking with Tom, but on the flagstand we had a rhythm that felt to me like magic. He motioned for me to give the 10-laps-to-go hand signal, then the five-to-go signal, and again I helped finish the white-flag lap before he took over in time to wave Shane Hmiel home for the win.

I had never been dirtier in my life than after that race. The dirt particles were light and felt like a mist. All my life I'd needed to feel clean—don't forget, avoiding dirty oil changes motivated me to help Frankie Neidenbach wave the flags—but I wore this dirt proudly.

The next night, I arrived at Indianapolis Raceway Park

with none of the trepidation I'd brought with me to Terre Haute or the Fairgrounds. I parked beside Tom's pickup, which had an IndyCar logo in the rear window. I smiled at that, wondering if someday I'd have something like that on my car. I grabbed my radio from the USAC hauler, where people were now saying, "Hello, Aaron." This was strange for me, but I took it as a sign that I hadn't screwed up and put myself at risk of being fired before I really got started.

That night, Tom let me wave the flags over some cars in qualifying. Again, the chills reached every cell inside me. When qualifying was over, I turned and spotted my dad in the grandstands. I'm fairly confident he had tears in his eyes. I know I did.

The racing that evening was intense, as pavement Midget racing tends to be, and at the start of the feature a car got launched over the backstretch wall and hit a Cadillac. I'm not sure how the policy reads, but it probably wasn't a good week for USAC's insurance carrier.

On the restart, a couple of laps in, I thought I saw a car throw heavier-than-normal sparks going into turn one. I reached to tap Tom to tell him, but if *I* wondered whether I'd really seen that, how could I explain it over the roar of 24 midgets? I reached for the radio button, but held my tongue again because, well, what would I say? The next lap, that car's right-rear tire went down at the same spot on the track, then spun into the wall. I vowed that from then on, I'd say something, and not question myself.

When Tom waved the twin checkered flags, I fought back tears. These had been the three most incredible days of my life. At the base of the stand, my dad and a friend from Massachusetts who was in town to attend the 500 were waiting for me. I shook Tom Hansing's hand; he had to get home and grab some sleep, because he was working the 500 the next day.

My dad was talking with a local flagman, and I overheard

him mentioning my aspirations of one day flagging the Indy 500. The man said, "Well, if he hangs out with Tom and does a good job, that's the way to the 500!"

Perhaps it was, but at that moment I looked up one last time to the stand that I had been working in, fearing that this was all there was and that I'd never get the chance again.

—— In the Shadow of the Pagoda ——

THE FOOTPRINT OF MY PRESENTATIONS ON AUTISM NOW covered all of Missouri, with several long trips across the state in June. But I had to admit that my mind had been elsewhere, knowing that I was scheduled to flag an event at the Indianapolis Motor Speedway in July. I wasn't kidding myself though; the Battle at the Brickyard for Quarter Midgets was not the Indianapolis 500, and, in fact, would not utilize any part of the 2.5-mile oval. Instead, it would take place on a track laid out in an infield parking lot, with a lap of less than one-tenth of a mile. But this was still the Indianapolis Motor Speedway.

When the weekend finally arrived, I got there early. The sun hadn't yet made its first appearance on the horizon when I made the left-hand turn off 16th Street and into the Speedway, passing under the "short chute" straightaway that connects turns one and two. I had made that turn numerous times to visit the museum, and it was surreal to do it as an employee of a racing series competing there.

It took me a bit to find the people I needed to meet, but I eventually met up with James Spink, who introduced me to Rick and Denise Thomason, the husband-and-wife race director and scorekeeper. They asked about my past experience, and I said that I had never seen a Quarter Midget race or flagged an oval-track event. I was honest, but I think this was a surprise to Rick, who turned to James and asked, "Really?"

But I felt like I was ready. Flagging my first race at Indianapolis was going to feel like taking a tightrope walk over the Grand Canyon, but one way to lessen the nerves was to be prepared. I'd read the rulebook many times, focusing on procedures and situations unique to oval-track racing. The vocabulary was different, with terms unfamiliar to me, but that's often the case when you move from one series to another.

The cars are called Quarter Midgets because they're exactly that, one-fourth the size of a full USAC-style Midget. But as soon as I waved the green flag, I understood that there was nothing small about the racing; it was as intense as anything I'd ever seen.

The class for the youngest drivers always got onto the track first. Looking back, it's interesting that among the kids in that event was 5-year-old Jake Garcia, who climbed the ladder to the NASCAR Truck Series. The speeds in that class were low, but there was action everywhere, and that was also true in the faster categories.

One thing I noticed immediately was that in Quarter Midgets, you can often hear the squeal of slipping tires over the engine noise. That kept me constantly looking around, thinking that perhaps a car was spinning. Occasionally, a driver would cut through the infield, as if he or she had gotten lost. I had never seen anything quite like this.

Practice came and went, and it was time for heat races. Getting the youngest kids off to a good, clean start was like trying to herd cats; they're so eager to race that it's tough to keep them aligned on their pace laps. Once we got to the 6-8-year-olds, things were more organized.

In the heats, drivers accumulated "passing points"—one

of those terms I'd never heard—that factored into where they would start in their features. I was astounded at how many passes there were a lap; if you blinked, you missed four overtaking moves. I'd never have believed that the lead could change in every turn of every lap, but I witnessed this in several heats.

With each event, my footing more secure, and the terms on the radio grew clearer. One thing that was *very* clear was James's desire to keep the show moving. There was one start I didn't quite like, so I waved it off, and immediately I heard James on the radio: "Aaron, there was *no reason* that was bad. Go green, stay green!"

Quarter Midgets are open-wheel machines, and sometimes when they touched wheels the crashes were huge. But these cars were definitely sturdy. I watched them flip, barrel roll, and slam into each other, and even after a nasty tumble, the car would be tipped back onto its wheels and stay in the race. The level of safety was impressive.

On the second day, something happened that I *still* haven't figured out. There were just two cars left in the heat race for the AA class, the fastest division at the time for the oldest kids. After they took the white flag, both cars slowed to a caution-flag pace as they exited turn two. I had no idea what was going on. I knew that each car was equipped with a RACEceiver, a one-way communication system over which the race director could alert the drivers when necessary; had they mistakenly been told that the yellow flag was out? When the cars completed the lap, I stood there frozen. I did not display the checkered flag. Confusion now reigned.

The USAC rules were clear about the idea that a race isn't over until the checkered flag falls. It is the law of all laws. If the checkered comes out a lap early or a lap late, the race is over at that point. Well, this race had not had a checkered flag. The two drivers continued slowly around the track, awaiting direction. James radioed, "Aaron, where was the checkered?"

I could only be honest. "They quit racing," I said. "I didn't know what to do." But the race distance had been met. The race director stopped the cars, and it was decided that the lap of the white flag would be considered the end, and then they had me display the checkered.

Fearing a harsh firing the likes of which had never been seen at the Speedway, I meekly packed my flags at the end of the day. I headed towards Rick and James to apologize. Even though the results of that heat race changed nothing, I felt like I'd let everyone down.

The next day, nothing was said about that incident, but I'd already relived it 10,000 times. I hadn't yet learned how to move on from mistakes. Sometimes I'm not sure I *ever* learned it. But it's an important skill, because for me a single mistake can make things rocky for days.

Fortunately, my last day flagging at the Battle at the Brickyard went well. During a break, I spoke with James's right-hand man, Kyle McCain. He complimented my work and asked if I'd be doing the remaining races in the USAC Quarter Midget series. I said I didn't know, but I took that as a good sign.

I had lived out a lifelong dream by flagging at the Indianapolis Motor Speedway. It wasn't the 500, but I waved the flags for that event like it was. Yet I worried, as usual, that this was it. I wish my brain didn't go to extremes like this, but once something is over, I always think it's over forever. My dad knew how I was thinking; he was watching from at home on the Internet stream, and he said he could see it in the way I somberly rolled up the flags.

But there was a surprise in store on my drive home to St. Louis. Even before I reached Terre Haute, James Spink called to ask if I'd work the Quarter Midget race at Eldora Speedway in Ohio later in the year. So, if the Battle at the Brickyard was an audition, I had passed.

I did the Eldora race, and then James asked if I wanted to flag the whole 2011 season. Just like that, I went from working just a few events per year to scheduling well over 20. Between racing and my presentations, I was going to be awfully busy. Life was good.

The Juggle

MANAGING MY TIME BECAME A DIFFICULT TASK. TOUCHPOINT Autism Services was getting requests from all over Missouri for my presentations, and there was no shortage of blog material from everyday life and the races I'd be working. My first USAC event of 2011 was in Phoenix, once again working with Rick, Denise, James, and Kyle. I'd quickly learn that, when working a 17-race calendar, the racing family becomes an extension of a real family.

The first real juggle came right before Phoenix, because I was the keynote presenter at a conference for Washington University's Intellectual and Developmental Disabilities Research Center in St. Louis. This was my biggest stage yet. Keynoting brings pressure and expectations; it's like starting on the front row of the Indy 500. And speaking of that, I was told that renowned researcher Dr. John Constantino would be seated in the front row while I spoke.

My heart was in my throat; I worried that Dr. Constantino might shoot down all of my abstract concepts. But as my presentation ended, I allowed myself for the first time to look in his direction, and he was the first one on his feet, giving me a standing ovation. Sadly, I had no time to bask in the glory, because I was out the door, hurrying to catch my flight to Phoenix.

In the morning, Kyle's alarm rang far too early. He said, "It's time to go, Liketens," adding a "t" to my name because he'd heard an announcer mispronounce it that way. It was still an hour before my alarm was set to go off, and I realized what happened: In Phoenix, daylight savings isn't a thing; they never move their clocks forward or backward. This was before smartphones automatically adjusted to local time zones, so when Kyle and James reset their phones to what they thought was Phoenix time, they got it wrong. I protested that I ought to get another hour of sleep, but they said I'd have to find my own way to the track. Off to the track we went, arriving while it was still dark. We were the only ones on the grounds.

That evening, a major life event occurred. I'd never gone out to eat with several of the USAC people, and they chose a Mexican restaurant. I'd never eaten Mexican food, but Denise said, "Aaron, if you want to work in racing, you've got to eat Mexican." I wasn't sure how the two things correlated, but in the door we went.

I was one of the pickiest eaters in the world, which is why I never went to dinner with others. I was close to a panic, but I figured this restaurant would have *something* I liked.

On the menu, the first words I saw were "steak burrito." Well, I liked steak, so that's what I ordered. When it came to the table, Denise and another scorer, Connie, were the first to see the agony on my face. Why? It had all the foods *touching* each other. In my own little world, the different foods on the plate were kept separate, not allowed to intermingle. I didn't know that in a burrito, everything was together *inside* the tortilla. And on the plate, the burrito was touching the lettuce, touching the beans, and touching the rice. This was a plate of chaos!

By now, everyone at the table was looking at me. James said something like, "Come on, bud, it'll be good for you!"

I had to eat, so slowly I brought the fork up to my mouth, ate my first bite of Mexican food, and thought … Where has *this* been all my life? *I liked it.* Mexican became the norm on our USAC trips.

Stories like that filled the year, and Ron Ekstrand was right about the blogging. Readers seemed to love my stories because they reflected obvious growth as I pushed my comfort zone outward. It was tiring, however. It was nothing to have a presentation in Springfield, Missouri, then make the *long* drive to Indy to ride with the USAC crew to a race in Michigan or Ohio.

But the biggest moment of 2011 came close to home, in St. Louis. Without my knowledge, I was registered to speak at a conference. When I first saw a flyer for the conference, I looked at the list of speakers and saw, right beside my own name, these three words: *Dr. Temple Grandin.* Just five years earlier, seeing Dr. Grandin speak was an absolute inspiration for me. Now we were together on a panel. Amazing.

It was also during 2011 that someone working for a division of Penguin Publishing discovered my blog and asked if I wanted to review a book. I said yes but added a twist: I told them that I had self-published a book of my own, and that I'd send them my book if they sent me one of theirs. There was no objection, and within a couple of months I had an offer for them to publish *Finding Kansas.* This was unbelievable! The book would be scheduled for release the following April.

I also had some flagging opportunities with USAC aside from the Quarter Midget series. I worked as a starter and assistant starter for events at Kalamazoo Speedway in Michigan, the Indianapolis Speedrome, and Columbus Motor Speedway in Ohio. Whether I was assisting Tom Hansing or working solo, it was all a treat.

When Donald Davidson told my dad that the path to the Indy 500 might be an apprenticeship with USAC, he suggested that the pay, if any, might be low, and the miles long. What he didn't mention was the camaraderie that would form. The long miles on the road got me to open up more, and the fun factor was high. Even if I often got back to St. Louis with the sun rising behind me, if this were the pathway to Indy, it would all be worth it.

Growth in Circles

THE PEOPLE I WORKED WITH IN BOTH SERIES—TONY LEONE at SKUSA and James and Kyle at USAC—loved getting me to step outside my comfort zone, whether by choice or by prank. At Newton Park in Lakeville, Indiana, they were going to appoint me tech director for the weekend unless I did some planking, a fad at the time. I knew nothing about engines or other technical matters, so I planked over a barrel of fuel. I have the photo to prove it.

Whether we were attending a roller derby in Kalamazoo, *walking* through a North Carolina drive-thru at midnight, checking into hotels at 3:00 a.m., or enduring a WKRP theme song marathon in Milwaukee, there was never a bad day. Meanwhile, I learned how intense some racing parents could be; one tried to pull me out of my flagstand when he disagreed with a call. It was interesting to see these parents look at each other, and sometimes scream at each other. And seeing the thrill of victory and the agony of defeat in kids and parents alike was part of the job.

Sometimes, the pranks would go too far. At a hotel in Ohio, Kyle had the front-desk person call repeatedly to say they were getting complaints about too much noise coming from my room. The joke in this was that I always had the quietest of rooms. At the time, I didn't see the humor, and I may have *overreacted* by just a hair—or a million hairs—when the desk clerk threatened to throw me out of the hotel. Only later, when I wrote a blog post about this episode, did I laugh at both the prank *and* my humorless attitude in the middle of it.

Working both the SKUSA SuperNats and USAC Battle at the Brickyard made me one of the nation's most prolific young flaggers. I loved where I was at, and even though the pay was absurdly low back then, it was nice on top of what I was earning by touring Missouri, making my presentations.

Racing is Dangerous as the Hits Keep Coming

THE YEAR 2012 BROUGHT THE RERELEASE OF *FINDING Kansas*, and a coast-to-coast book tour in conjunction with World Autism Month. Just a week before the tour was set to begin, the USAC Generation Next tour had its second race of the year, held in Nashville. The previous year there, it was so bitterly cold that even doing my best Michelin Man impression thanks to all the layers I was wearing, the cold still pierced to the bone.

Weather played a role in 2012 as well; Saturday rains meant we were always a bit behind schedule, but Sunday had bright, sunny skies. The racing had been rough and tumble all day, but with 18 laps to go in the feature for what is called the Junior Animal class, things got really intense. We were coming off a yellow-flag slowdown, and the public-address speakers were blaring the song "Don't Stop Believing" by Journey. I remember that very clearly.

I threw the green flag for the restart, and the field was just completing that lap when the leader spun exiting turn four. I waved the yellow, and a handful of cars made it past the spinning car before it stopped. I could see what came next before the drivers could. Two cars were side-by-side, and the driver on the inside was moving to his right to avoid that stopped car. But in doing so, he touched the car to his outside, and the two cars made contact with the Tecpro barrier on the frontstretch, just short of the flagstand.

Now, I must point out that the flagstand at Nashville couldn't have been more dangerous. It was a free-standing structure outside a curving frontstretch with a movable temporary wall just in front of it. Sure, I use strong words now, but on that day, I wasn't going to let logic and safety stop me from my job. I wish I had.

The two cars started to push the Tecpro into the flagstand. I could see it all happening, but I was powerless to stop it, so I just kept waving the yellow. The barrier was pushed back against the stand and seemed to release its energy in all directions. The car that struck the wall hardest flipped violently; I was first flung forward and almost out of the stand onto the track, then fell backwards and almost out the back of the stand. Instead, I sank to the floor of the stand, but the damage had already been done.

I remember looking up at the sky. Much like my first big kart crash, the pain didn't start until I tried to breathe. I screamed, silently, as I had no breath. "Don't stop … believing…" repeated over and over before the song was interrupted by the announcer's voice over the speakers: "We need medical to the flagstand. Medical to the flagstand, please."

Above me, I heard voices asking if I was all right. The first person to me was Debi Supan, USAC's PR representative. I remember that she had a guitar around her neck;

all the winners in Nashville got a guitar as a trophy, and she'd been waiting to hand this one out. I tried to speak but couldn't.

I was hurting in numerous places. What kept me from falling out of the stand was that my left ankle had gotten caught by a metal crossbeam, injuring both the ankle and shin. There was no doubt that I was going to the hospital. There were concerns that the ankle might be broken, as well as my hip and some ribs. But my neck and back were fine, so instead of waiting for an ambulance I was loaded into a car. One man who helped in this process was Paul Lushin, who was there with his racing son. Paul co-owned the Derek Daly Academy, so technically I'd worked for him back in 2003. Trying to make me feel better, Paul said, "Aaron, it hurts now, but this is building your legacy for when you make it to Indy." All I wanted was to breathe without feeling like a broadsword was cutting my insides. The races went on after I was driven away.

A racer's mom went with me to the hospital, and I guess as soon as they gave me the heavy pain meds, I became a real chatterbox, and then an emotional wreck. I know I was worried about my book tour the following week. This was not the time to get smoked in the stand.

After a couple of hours, my x-rays and test results were all in. I had some cracked ribs and a bruised pelvis, plus a sprained ankle and two hematomas forming on my shins. The doctor said that aside from a strong ache during deep breaths, I should have no problems doing my tour.

When I got back to the track, the day's races were over. But James said he had something for me; I was given one of the winners' guitars, my first trophy in quite some time. I just wish I hadn't had to crack some bones to earn it.

The doctor was right: I had no issues with my tour, which got off to a good start.

My next racing job was the SKUSA SpringNationals kart

race in Phoenix. That track had an enclosed flagstand, and in one of the junior events there was a tangle on the start. One kart spun, stopped, and was hit by another one, which started tumbling toward me. That kart's nose came to rest on the ledge of my stand.

I may not have been gun-shy before, but I was starting to get that way. At the Orange Show Speedway in San Bernardino, California—a race that aligned with the book tour—I saw the underside of a Quarter Midget headed my way. Thankfully, it stayed on the correct side of the fence, but it was one more incident to think about. Was it open season on Aaron Likens?

Finally, on June 1, at Grundy County Speedway in Morris, Illinois, I had a race without a serious incident. And it was a big night for me, my first time working solo in a USAC National Midget Series race, which I considered another career milestone. What made it even better was that my dad was able to attend.

But next time out, at Little Kalamazoo Speedway, things went bad again.

That's one of those places where everything happens fast. The quickest Quarter Midgets turn laps in less than five seconds. I repeat: *less than five seconds.*

In one of the finals, the last-place driver spun as the leaders were closing in to lap him. It happened right in front of me, almost at my feet. As at Nashville, I could see what was going to happen before the drivers did. Some of the drivers were unsighted, blocked from seeing the spun car because they were in traffic; inevitably, one kid hit it, launching his car straight up and into the corner of the flagstand. Thankfully, whoever built it made it extremely strong, but the impact still blasted me backward and out of the stand, and the impact with the ground knocked me out. The next thing I knew, I was in an ambulance, being asked if I wanted morphine. I don't know how I responded, but I know I was given the morphine.

The X-rays came back negative, and Kyle McCain, who was in the process of taking over as director of the series, came to pick me up at the hospital. I was loopy from the morphine and therefore not responding clearly to the questions asked of me, so the docs didn't know if they should release me yet. At this point, into the ER came an ambulance crew with a couple of people who'd been in a passenger car crash. Kyle turned around and saw a person who was not in good shape being wheeled by on a gurney. Kyle's face became flushed. He said, "I'm never going to forget that, Liketens."

Well, it's not like I wanted to be there, either!

Eventually I was released, and from there I have no memory, although Kyle filled me in later. We got back to the USAC office in Indianapolis at 4:00 a.m., and although Kyle said I could stay with him, I insisted on driving home to St. Louis. My next memory is of waking up in the back of my car in a rest area on I-70, somewhere west of Indy, having changed into my sleeping clothes and made a nice bed for myself. I had no memory of driving there, parking the car, or changing my clothes.

All of these dramas meant that I had no lack of things to write about in my blog, but getting bruised and injured was getting tiresome. I had been hurt more times flagging races than driving in them, a fact not lost on my mom. She said, "Remember when I told you to stop driving and just flag? I think I regret saying that."

She suggested that I maybe should "quit this racing stuff," but I was too invested. I thought of my life with racing and without racing, and I couldn't see myself happy without it. From the F1 atmosphere of the SKUSA Super-Nats in Las Vegas to the all-American vibes at places like the Quarter Midget track in Hagerstown, Maryland, I loved it, and I wasn't ready to give it up.

When My Two Worlds Met

THROUGHOUT 2012, MY PRESENTATION SCOPE INCREASED. Sadly, Matt's state funding ended in 2011, so I was no longer doing the lunch-and-learn sessions at doctors' offices, but I learned I could be highly effective, and entertaining, at schools. It didn't start out all that great, though; my first school presentation late in 2011 was to a class of fifth-grade kids, and going into it I was more nervous than I'd been for any other presentation I'd done.

The morning of the presentation, I called Ron and begged him not to have me do this. I mean, what could I possibly say that a fifth grader would understand? Please don't think I'm selling kids short. My nervousness stemmed from a complete lack of confidence in my words when facing a new audience. Did I have to change my stories? My examples? What did I have to do to not completely bomb? But the presentation was a must, so I tried to make the best of it.

My coworker, Jennifer, introduced me. As I took to the front of the classroom, I couldn't help thinking I was back in Mrs. Colvin's class, asked to give a book report but unable to speak.

By this point, I had given a couple hundred presentations, but suddenly I was back to the year 1991. I could not say a word, not even my name. It was awkward. It was painful. After the longest 15 seconds of my life, having 25 young humans staring at me in disbelief, I turned to the teacher and whispered "help." She spoke up and said, "Mr. Likens, why don't you begin by telling us what autism is." That was a good idea, so I pointed with my index finger up, to signal one. But … one what? What one thing could I tell these kids about autism?

At about this time, a kid in the center of the class either knew the answer or wanted to end this awkward situation, so he raised his hand. He said, "Excuse me, Mr. Likens, but if I'm not mistaken, isn't autism simply that you see and process the world around you differently?"

What an excellent answer! It's been one of my opening lines in school presentations since that day. The rest of the presentation flowed naturally. I've been amazed at how kids can grasp the essence of the autism spectrum. Even kindergartners, probably the most intimidating audiences I've faced, somehow instantly understand sensory issues.

Schools became a main focus, and I was now speaking to thousands of people a month. Because of this, I was honored as one of three individuals named a "Mental Health Champion" by the Missouri Department of Mental Health.

In May of 2012, I wanted to do a video blog in recognition of the man who set all this in motion: Duane Sweeney. I wanted to record it in Duane's "office," the flagstand of the Indianapolis Motor Speedway. My dad made a few calls and got in touch with Doug Boles. Today, Doug is president of IMS, but in 2012 he was its head of marketing. My dad told Doug the story of Duane giving me a signed checkered flag, about my racing career, and about what I'd done with my book and presentations.

Doug's answer to the idea was, "Absolutely!"

We were given an awesome date to do this: the day before the 2012 Indianapolis 500. Arriving at the track and picking up our credentials was a new and exciting experience. It was hard not to imagine what this would feel like on race day and going to the flagstand to work.

My first time at the base of the flagstand's narrow ladder was intimidating. It seemed to stretch all the way to heaven, and, to me, it did. I didn't know I had a fear of heights until I got about halfway up, but once I was in the flagstand itself, I felt nothing but elation. This was it, the exact spot I'd thought so much about. Would I ever get the chance to stand here with cars on track? If I did, the long days, the hours, the broken bones … it would all be worth it.

But I wasn't there to daydream. My dad got the microphone and camera ready, and I delivered a heartfelt thanks to Duane for giving me the item—that signed flag—that deepened my passion for racing. Without that flag, there would've been no book, no self-confidence, no presentations to help others; I couldn't imagine what my life would have been like. The premise of the video was to encourage everyone to be nicer, and perhaps mentor a person on the autism spectrum because there's no way to know the magnitude of what that might lead to.

When I finished, my dad had a tear in his eye. Behind him, Doug Boles was full of emotion. He told me that my words hit home because his dad had been a caretaker of sorts for Duane in his final years at the Speedway.

As we exited the stand, Doug said he got to choose an honorary starter for a day of practice for the 500, so for the following year he'd see what he could do.

Nearly a year later, in the spring of 2013, I was driving on the backroads of Missouri—I remember the exact spot, between Vienna and Iberia—when I got a phone call from my dad. He started with, "Aaron, I need to read you an email." Then the phone went *beep, beep, beep* … A dropped call.

He called back and said that the email was from Doug Boles, and … *beep, beep, beep* …

Well, I had waited my entire life for the opportunity that I hoped this email might bring, so what was a few extra seconds?

Finally, my cell signal improved enough for my dad to read Doug's email. It said that for my advocacy on behalf of autism and my work as a speaker and author, I'd been invited to wave the green flag for a day of practice leading up to the 2013 Indianapolis 500.

I'd be fulfilling a dream, and maybe a destiny assigned to me when Duane Sweeney gave me that checkered flag.

—— A Lifetime's Wait for a Single Car ——

MAY 13, 2013, WAS THE DAY I'D GET TO STAND ATOP A platform on the Indianapolis Motor Speedway pit wall and wave the green flag to start a day of practice. The platform would be close to the spot where the late Pat Vidan used to wave the flags in the days when the official starter was stationed at the edge of the track. That bit of history only added to the anticipation that made the evening of May 12 seem like the longest of my life.

Despite the lack of real sleep, I felt nothing but joy in my heart as we headed to the Speedway. It was a brisk and windy morning. I worried if any cars would bother taking to the track. Wouldn't it be disappointing to get this opportunity, and then have to wave the flag over an empty track?

My dad has a skill for talking his way past anyone. The Speedway's yellow-shirted security staffers kept pointing us toward a parking area inside turn four, but he convinced them all that we needed to be right next to the track's famous pagoda.

I brought my own green flag. I'd seen the track's flag, which had a longer dowel, and it looked too heavy for my waving style. If this turned out to be my only chance to wave a green flag on the frontstretch at Indianapolis, I wanted a wave I'd be happy with for the rest of my life.

The hour of noon drew near. The platform was placed, a waiver signed, and a PR man walked me across the pit lane. It was one of the most intimidating walks of my life. The empty grandstands seemed to be closing in. I looked across the track and saw Tom Hansing in the flagstand. He smiled and shouted, "Aaron, don't drop it!"

Great, I wasn't thinking about dropping the flag until then.

The PR man came back with the official green flag and was confused when he saw that I was already holding one.

He asked, "You're using that one?" He took it from me and inspected it the way a craftsman would inspect his finished work. My flag passed, and it was just about noon.

The PR man had a radio, and I was watching Tom. The seconds to the top of the hour ticked agonizingly slowly. But then I heard the call, "green flag, starter, green flag," and Tom pointed down at me. My green flag flew in the air and … there was no engine noise. Nothing. But then an engine came to life, and JR Hildebrand took to the track. There was only one taker, but at least I'd have the chance to wave a green to a race car.

Hildebrand's car came into sight off of turn four, and I confidently raised the flag. When it came down, I improvised a bit with my style, and swooshed the flag across my body as the car crossed the line. A still photo later showed that I'd replicated the pose Pat Vidan used when flagging there. And with Hildebrand's car speeding past me, the moment was over. As I climbed from the platform, I heard public-address announcer Dave Calabro say, "Smile, Aaron, it's okay. There it is, and what a smile!"

Tom Surber wrote a very nice story for the IMS website about my day as honorary starter, and about my work as a presenter, author, and advocate. There was one line in that article that gave me hope: "His ultimate dream is to be the flagman at the Indianapolis 500," Tom wrote, "and he's taking all the necessary steps to make that happen."

My chance to wave the green at Indy was done. I hoped Indy wasn't done with me.

And what became of the green flag I used that day? Properly, it rests right next to the checkered flag Duane Sweeney gave me.

The People I Worked With

IT WAS NICE BEING CONGRATULATED BY MY RACING COWORKERS on my honorary-starter day at the Speedway. My routine for 2013 again involved SKUSA and USAC, and the people I knew best with both of those series continued to help me expand my limits.

James Spink started to take more of a hands-off role with the Quarter Midgets—which USAC called its .25 Midget series—and Kyle McCain began to step in as the next series director. James wasn't done with me, though; he'd take me to restaurants where he knew the foods on the plate would be touching, or where the staff was loud, because he knew that certain types of noise still bothered me. James and other USAC people tested me in ways that were fun, but not over the top. They also helped me build the confidence to speak up. There were times with James, and also with Terry Bybee of SKUSA, when we walked into restaurants that had live bands, and each time I stopped in the doorway and said, "This isn't going to work for me." Self-advocating in that way is a hard thing for me to do, but because those guys knew about autism and my challenges, I felt comfortable speaking up.

Across Missouri, my coworkers started booking presentations that matched my strengths. As nice as they all were to me, I'm sure I was often blank in return; I use "blank" because I don't know a better word. I appreciated what everyone was doing for me, and I especially appreciated the friendship, but it was a one-way street, which can be the case with someone on the autism spectrum. It wasn't that I didn't like them, but I had no idea how to show it, say it, or even acknowledge it. A wall separates the part of my brain that appreciates these things from the part of my brain that fails to find the words.

One morning when I was getting ready for a SKUSA

event in Lancaster, California, I got a phone call from someone at TouchPoint, letting me know that Matt Schafer had suddenly passed away.

Matt and I had done so many presentations together, and he had allowed me to be the star in those sessions. In the end, that may have cost him his job. His position was funded by a grant and when the funding ran out, TouchPoint kept him on for a while. The time came, however, when he was let go. Maybe the thinking was: Why fund the wingman to the person the doctors and nurses wanted to speak to? But if not for Matt, I might never have had the confidence to present in a competent manner. On my flight to California, I wrote a eulogy of sorts with sentences such as:

"I always thought this had to be hard for Matt. He made the contact, he set up the meeting, and then I became the star. In one of these meetings, a doctor literally pushed Matt out of the way so she could talk to me more. He always took this in stride, though, and often joked about it."

To finish, I wrote:

"As much as I didn't want to write this, I don't want to finish it. To finish this, in a way, is my final goodbye, and how do I say it? How do I say goodbye to the person who helped hone my craft? I might have burned out, flamed out, or became frustrated with myself and may never have gotten to the point where I am now. I mean, I'm about to start my second national tour, and when I started out in 2010 that wasn't something that was even imaginable. So how do I say goodbye, knowing I never really thanked him? Perhaps I can't, as nothing would be fitting. So instead of me coming up with a way to finish this dedication, I'll let his words finish it. Matt sent this to me right before my national tour last year. He hadn't worked at TouchPoint for almost a year, but autism was still on his mind. Here's what he sent me:

"'Aaron … I know you haven't heard from me since I left TouchPoint, but I heard something good, and I thought you

could use it. A week or so ago, a parent of a young man told me, 'Folks with autism will change the world because the world can't change them. The world can't change you, Aaron, and you will change the world.'

Goodbye, Matt. Thank you for helping me become who I am. In every presentation I give, I'll remember that I wouldn't be who I am without you."

I didn't know how, but I vowed to try and actually connect with those that I work with. I don't think I've ever done a good job with that, and it's one of the major regrets I have in my life. But those I've worked with, who have understood me, they knew—or at least I hope they knew—that they meant everything to me, even though I may have been stoic, quiet, and seemingly indifferent.

The Most Difficult Race

ASK ANYONE IN RACING ABOUT THE MOST DIFFICULT WEEKEND they've ever had, and I'm sure they can name at least one where nothing seemed to go right. For myself, the answer is obvious: the Streets of Modesto event from the SKUSA Pro Tour of 2014.

It was summertime in California's San Joaquin Valley. The air seemed to not move at all, and the daytime temperature was 112 degrees. The race organizers, familiar with the local weather, had scheduled a night race, which might make for a great spectacle under the lights.

When practice began on Friday, the first group of karts didn't make it two laps before the red flag was out for a crash. This set the tempo for the next 30 hours or so. A typical kart track has large runoff areas, in some cases 100 feet of dirt or grass between a fast corner and anything solid. On street circuits like Modesto, that's not possible; the course is lined with walls, usually on both sides. But for some reason, many of the drivers ran the fast Modesto track as if the walls didn't exist and they had all the runoff room in the world.

When racing started on Saturday, the crashes got severe. These weren't typical kart crashes; these were brutal, savage. I lost count of the number of times the red flag flew that day, but 35 seems to be the consensus among folks who were there. The event was supposed to consist of two complete SKUSA programs, one Saturday and one Sunday, but as the crashing continued into the night on Saturday, that almost didn't seem possible.

From my vantage point, I could not see the carnage taking place around the track. This was a street circuit, so buildings obscured the view of the .88-mile track.

By their nature, most street circuits include endless 90-degree corners. The Modesto layout was different; the final corner of the lap, turn 12, was a quick right-left flick, almost a sweeping chicane. I had a good view of that area, and despite all the crashing elsewhere, there had been no incidents in this right-left complex. But sometime after dark, one kart clipped the barrier at the exit of turn 12 and was sent into a spin. The drivers right behind him didn't have much time to react, nor any runoff, and no less than eight karts piled in at full speed. It was sickening to watch. I jumped down from my platform, fearing the worst for some of the drivers.

Sprinting to the scene, I radioed Terry, the race director, recommending "full-course yellow" as the track was almost blocked. As I got there, the drivers were rising from their karts. Checking each one quickly, I assessed that there were no injuries of significance. Again, I radioed, "Terry, are we full-course yellow?" There wasn't a response, but since I had radioed twice, I felt confident we were.

As I started to pull a kart out of the groove, I looked up and a corner worker was standing right beside me, staring at me. It was at that moment I heard it: the roar of a finely tuned shifter-kart engine at speed. At speed. One of two things was happening; either the leader was ignoring the full-course yellow, or—and this would be a disaster—we were *not* full-course yellow!

I screamed at the worker, "Where's your flag?" He didn't know. I had an 80-percent-blocked track, exposed barriers, drivers standing in dangerous places, and no warning flags. I ran toward turn 11, screaming into my radio, "YELLOW! TURN 11! YELLOW, PLEASE!" The chicane, turn 12, was almost blind on entry and the coming drivers would not be expecting a kart in the center of the track, or people standing around.

I began leaping in the air to be seen, and to convey the severity of the situation. I was way too close to the groove, but I was hoping to avoid a series of 60 MPH impacts. As the dense pack of karts went past me, still racing, I prayed an informal prayer out loud, "God, no, please no …" I feared the sickening sound of the impact I was assured was coming. When the last kart passed me, I slowly turned my head back toward turn 12 and was shocked. No other karts had crashed. Why? Because the drivers who'd been in the pileup, realizing what was about to happen, quickly pitched in to clear the track.

Just then, I heard Terry radio, "Aaron, what's this about a yellow in 11?"

We pieced it all together later, and what happened was this: When I'd taken off running from the flagstand to turn 12, calling Terry to say that we needed a full-course yellow, he was calling me to see if the track was clear. Our two radio calls basically cancelled each other out. When I tried again a moment later, Terry was doing the same thing. I assumed that he heard me, and he assumed that I heard him. I thought we had a full-course yellow, and Terry thought we had a clear track. The lesson here was: Until you hear the word "copy," or a read-back of your radio call, *never* assume that your message got through.

Several hours later, at a little before 1:00 a.m., there was a violent crash on the back side of the track. During the red flag, driver after driver walked past me at start/finish wearing serious faces; one driver, especially haunted by what he'd seen, shouted to announcer Rob Howden, "She's dead, I tell you. Dead. I'm done." Thankfully, the driver mentioned was not dead, and in fact every driver who crashed that night would recover.

The strangest incident of the event, and one of the oddest I've ever seen, came at just past 2:00 a.m., when we had a red flag for beer. Beer!

Getting set for another race, I walked toward the starting lights, and felt some drops of liquid as I passed beneath the pedestrian bridge. When I looked up, more drops hit the lenses of my glasses. I looked down, and at my feet was a growing puddle. Someone had dropped a beer—or, more likely, beers—on the bridge, and now we had a pool of beer in the braking zone for turn one. I called for a red, and delayed the start until we could soak up the suds.

At 2:58 a.m., I threw the final checkered flag of the night, and not a moment too soon, because there was 3:00 a.m. curfew.

We were back at it on Sunday morning, and thankfully everything went smoothly. The drivers respected the track and the speeds, the racing was clean, and the red flag made only a couple of inconsequential appearances.

I've never had another event like Modesto, and I'm not alone in that feeling. Ask anyone who was there, and you'll probably see them shudder. SKUSA is a great series with phenomenal racing, but sometimes you just have those days.

The Era of Kyle

WHEN KYLE MCCAIN BECAME THE FULL USAC .25 MIDGET series director, I sort of became a sounding board, because we spent dozens of hours in the car. Aside from James Spink moving on, the USAC .25 crew had remained the same, with Rick and Denise Thomason, and Butch Lamb, the announcer. There had been a revolving door of annual interns, and it was neat to see some of them move on in the sport, with Brent Butler making it to ThorSport Racing, a NASCAR Truck Series team, and Alex Offenbach joining Andretti Autosport in IndyCar before moving to other teams.

I probably spent more hours in the car with Kyle than I have with anyone else, family aside. I'd become part of another family as we traveled from town to town, working in youth motorsports. Whether playing Monopoly on the iPhone, or games of "would you rather," there was no shortage of laughter and camaraderie. One day, I was "forced" to spike my hair; it happened to be the same day our group acted up at Barefoot Bernies, a restaurant in Hagerstown, Maryland. Then there was the time Kyle may have or may not have inadvertently driven through a national park with two 55-gallon barrels of racing fuel. It was always an adventure, and while times at the track could be intense, we'd always end the weekend laughing at some absurdity we'd witnessed or commenting on how great the races had been.

In 2014, I spent two weeks on the road with Kyle when we remained out East between races in Hagerstown and New Castle, Delaware. In the week between, we stopped in Washington D.C. and went to several of the Smithsonian museums, then stayed in Baltimore and went to an Orioles game at Camden Yards. Through all the miles we drove, he somehow "got" me like few have, and each race was a treat to work.

At the end of 2014, we had a Christmas party in Indianapolis, and the activity we chose was indoor karting. The end result? At the finish line, Kyle got turned and I tried to avoid him on the right, but he clipped the rear of my kart, which sent me airborne. I went over the track wall and slammed into another wall; it was the hardest impact I've ever felt. Rick Thomason, who was behind me, hit my rear axle with his steering wheel as I ricocheted back onto the track. Rick had some serious hand injuries, and he was taken off to the hospital after instructing us to go to his house and act as if nothing major had occurred. So, Kyle and I went to their house, and we told Denise that Rick had been in "just a small crash, nothing to worry about." Why were we told not to tell the truth? The truth, whatever it was, would come out eventually.

Denise was upstairs when we heard her phone ring.

"You did *what*?" she screamed? "You lost *what*?" She came down the stairs and somehow didn't strangle the two of us. We both said, "Rick made us do it!" In the end, Rick lost a finger and part of another one.

I went to the doctor the next day and found out I had cracked my tailbone.

The high-flying era wasn't over. Our 2015 USAC season started for us in Huntsville, Alabama. In the very first heat race, two cars came together and slid toward the outside wall. A third car came in and ramped over the first two, and that car just flew. This Quarter Midget was almost eight feet in the air, and almost cleared the retaining fence.

I knew Kyle was in trouble. He was spotting in turn two, in a place that would've been safe in any instance but this one. As that airborne car bounced off the fence, it caught Kyle in the head, and from my vantage point he disappeared behind the wall with the car right on top of him.

The race was stopped, and I turned away. This was a crash far more severe than you expect in a Quarter-Midget event. We'd had drivers break a hand or a foot, injuries no worse than kids might get playing baseball or football in school, but this?

The driver was okay, but Kyle was not. I was not going to walk over to the scene. I was not going to check to see how he was doing. By the way the medical personnel were working diligently at the scene, I could only fear that Kyle was badly injured.

The flagstand was my friend. I didn't exit it. I looked the opposite way, trying to maintain my emotions. My friend had been hit in the head by a flying race car.

I don't remember who it was, but someone came over to me and simply said, "He's alive, and talking, and I think he laughed." I finally could breathe without forced labor. The ambulance left with Kyle, and at the start of the very next heat race, one car lost control and hit another in the right rear, hooking that second car into the flagstand. It was not a good day for officials.

My injury was minimal, a hematoma on my shin, but I stayed in the game. Kyle, on the other hand, had a head injury that bled quite a lot, and some foot injuries where the car had landed squarely. He had been a star athlete in high school, and his recovery was impressive.

Late that season, we had a most-embarrassing episode. I've been careful not to tell this story too many times, because I was partly to blame. We wrapped up a race outside Philadelphia and when we were done, we headed west towards Indianapolis. At the time, Alex, Kyle, and a USAC intern were constantly playing the iPhone version of *Sports Jeopardy!* I'd host. It was a great way to converse and kill time on a 700-mile journey. There was a fifth person in the vehicle, another intern, who didn't care for this at all, but he'd come into play the next day.

We were about three-quarters of the way to Pittsburgh when Kyle pulled off the highway and we checked into a hotel. The next morning, the *Jeopardy!* tournament continued.

The games were close, the smack talk was getting personal, and each game ended with someone shouting "rematch!" At some point, the intern not playing said, "Gettysburg? Didn't we see that sign yesterday?" Our hearts sank; we hadn't noticed that we'd been heading *east*, into the rising sun. Two hours east, plus two to get back to where we'd started, added four hours to our long drive.

Kyle departed USAC at the end of 2015. The final race we worked together was in Grand Rapids, Michigan, and it was emotional. I don't like change, and this was going to be a major one. James had hired me, and he'd left, and now it was Kyle leaving.

We had a final dinner with the original crew, and it was difficult thinking that this would be the last time we'd all be together. All the racing families I've been a part of have had this type of atmosphere, and it's painful when you know it's coming to an end. Sure, there's the "we'll stay in touch" discussion when you say goodbye, but there's nothing like going out on a race track and *knowing* they'll have your back no matter what happens.

The changing of the guard with the Quarter Midgets was a harbinger of what was ahead: the next saga of my life, and maybe the darkest years of my life.

—— The Last Bit of Joy Before the Pain ——

LIFE CAN PRESENT THE MOST RANDOM OF OPPORTUNITIES, AND the cryptic nature of this chapter's title is intentional, because this joy wasn't just joy, but rather another feeling of destiny.

It was May of 2016, and the first week of practice for the 100th running of the Indianapolis 500. I was at the Speedway to flag the EV Grand Prix, an event run in conjunction with Purdue University and USAC for university students who built and competed with battery-powered karts. It was one of the odder events I've ever experienced, not because of the technology but because of the drivers involved. Some teams had a driver who'd never raced before, and on another was a driver who competed in what is now called the Indy NXT series, which is the category right below IndyCar. The speed discrepancies were, well, dangerous. The fastest driver was lapping the slowest driver every two or three laps, and the distance from inside boundary to outside wall wasn't much more than two kart-widths. Lindy Thackston, an Indianapolis broadcast journalist, was upended when a kart hit a wall where she was standing.

The event was different, but I gave it my all because once again I was flagging at the Indianapolis Motor Speedway. We were using a lot in the infield, but I could hear the IndyCar drivers practicing on the oval, which allowed me to imagine I was over at the big flagstand.

Before the main event, Doug Boles, who was, by now, track president, walked over and asked me how it was going; he had a son competing in the high-school portion of the EV Grand Prix. Then Doug said, "Hey, when are you going back to St. Louis?" My ears perked up, and I replied, "That depends on what you mean by your question."

Doug said that Tom Hansing wouldn't be flagging the next day's practice sessions, and he was wondering if I might want to be in the stand. I asked him to repeat what he'd said, because I couldn't believe it. I smiled and said, "Absolutely!" Doug said that it was not a done deal, and that he would text me that evening to confirm.

The EVGP wrapped up, and for the rest of the day I checked my phone about every 10 seconds. By 10:00 p.m.,

I decided to give up and go to sleep hoping for something positive overnight. When I awoke, there still were no missed calls and no texts.

I left my sister Kimberly's condo on the north side of Indy around 11:00 a.m. Practice would start at noon, so I assumed Doug and IndyCar had made other plans. My idea was to grab a bite to eat and then head home. Sitting in the restaurant—a Noble Roman's on 10th Street—I had a notion: I never spoke up for myself, never chased after a job; I convinced myself that it was okay to text Doug to confirm that they had other plans, and to thank him for thinking of me in the first place.

I sent the text, and before I put the phone down, I saw that little three-dot icon indicating that he was texting back. He apologized for not staying in touch and told me to get to the track ASAP; he wanted me to stop at the credential office, pick up a silver badge, and meet him in the infield. I did all that, and there was a golf cart waiting for me. Doug was in the middle of a TV interview, but when that was finished, he took me up to race control, in the pagoda. Then we walked under the track, and I followed him to the stand I'd thought about forever.

I had climbed the ladder before, but it was still daunting. I could see the official flags waiting up there. With each rung of the ladder, I had flashbacks of being at the track when I was younger, and of the time I met Duane Sweeney. I thought of all the years, and the people I'd worked with. Even if this was just a one-day thing, my God, what an opportunity!

In the stand were a pit-road official filling in along with Jeff Boles, Doug's dad, known as Judge, because until he retired in 2014, that's what he'd been: a circuit court judge. Judge had worked in various roles at the Speedway since the early '60s. He gave me a headset tuned to hear the observers stationed around the track, and Doug asked if I needed anything.

"This is all I've ever wanted," I replied. "I'm perfectly fine."

And I stood in that flagstand with cars flashing beneath me at 230 miles per hour.

A few minutes later, Judge suddenly stomped his feet on the floor of the flagstand, a jolt that I could feel through my own feet and legs. Was he upset about something? Had I done something wrong? No, this was simply protocol. Whenever Judge heard through his headset that race control had called for a caution, he would stomp his feet as an unmistakable cue for his assistant to throw the yellow flag. He'd just forgotten to tell me.

When practice was set to resume, the other official on the stand handed me the green flag so I could get things officially restarted. Several cars pulled off pit road and onto the track. On my practice day in 2013, I waved the green for just one car; this time, it would be for a big group. I wasn't going to go overboard, but I sure as hell was going to make it look good.

Simon Pagenaud led the string of cars out of turn four, and my green flag fluttered in the springtime air at Indianapolis. My movements were precise, and as the last car passed, I smiled. No one would notice a green flag in a practice session, and no one *should* notice a green flag in a practice session, but I felt like I deserved this after the single-car green three years earlier.

Wait, did I say no one noticed? As I put the green flag back in its holder, I heard a noise and looked in the direction it was coming from. A closed-circuit TV camera attached to the top of the catch fence at the flagstand was squealing as it turned. Its lens was pointing towards the ground as it turned, but now it tilted upward to look at the flagstand. I tried moving out of its path, but the lens followed me. On my headset radio, I heard a woman's voice: "Race control would like to know who waved the flag."

Judge replied, "That would be Aaron Likens from St. Louis, Missouri, a tremendous starter in his own right!"

The lady in race control said, "Okay. Race control notes that it looked fantastic!"

I stayed on the stand for the remaining four hours or so of practice, watching and listening. I later learned that after I'd been up there a while, someone at race control, using a channel I could not hear, suggested that I leave; normally, guests on the flagstand don't stay so long. But the pit official who was filling in on the stand responded, "Look, he knows what he's doing, and I don't." That answer was what allowed me to experience the rest of the day.

Somehow, word was getting around among my friends that I was in the flagstand. My phone buzzed with texts of congratulations. Rob Howden, the SKUSA announcer, was working the pits for the Indianapolis Motor Speedway Radio Network; during a break in practice, he took a selfie at the yard of bricks with me in the background. Rob and I always talked about making it to Indianapolis, and at this moment, we were both there.

The official practice clock kept ticking down. Every 60 seconds, I was another minute closer to the end of this once-in-a-lifetime experience. Finally, my headset said, "One minute, starter." The official waved the checkered flag at 6:00 p.m., marking the end of practice, but then he handed it to me: a trio of cars, the last three practicing, exited turn four and headed down the front straightaway. Tears welled up in my eyes as I waved the checkered flag over them.

During breaks in practice, I had talked with Judge about Duane Sweeney, who had died in 2004. Now, with the day done, I said, "I'd give anything to be able to tell Duane about this, and that I am the person I am because of his flag."

My car was parked by the track office outside turn one. I was walking through the parking lot when Doug Boles came out and shook my hand. He said the flag waving looked amazing. I was choked up, fighting off tears. I thanked him profusely, but I was unable to tell him that this was the best day of my life, the best experience of my life.

Nor could I put into words the sadness I felt because this wonderful experience was over. I mean, what were the odds that I'd ever get another chance to climb that flagstand?

The Loss of a Title

AFTER RON EKSTRAND LEFT THE ORGANIZATION WHERE I'd been working, I was reporting to a man named David. I was promised that the arrangements I'd had in place would remain; my blog was part of my job, and the time I spent going to races was considered work because it showed what a person on the autism spectrum could accomplish. This seemed like a smart idea, particularly after my one day of flagging practice at Indianapolis, but some of the new people I worked with were indifferent to this achievement. That was the first sign of a crack in the foundation.

Slowly, things started to change, and I was faced with things I didn't know how to handle. At a meeting about social-media engagement, I was asked by a marketing person why I didn't communicate with a coworker about something that was, in the big picture, quite trivial. I should have said it was because I was on the autism spectrum, so sometimes communication was complicated. But I didn't say that; in fact, I said nothing at all, and for an hour I faced a barrage of questions on this topic. I maintained my composure until the woman said, "Aaron, they're your coworkers, they're your friends, you can talk to them," and followed this with four words that pierced my heart: "It's not that difficult."

It's ... not ... that ... difficult.

Those words hit me unlike anything else in my life. You've read about the challenges I had at the workplace, and you've read about the heights I'd been able to reach. All of those heights were erased, and I was reduced to one sentence. I allowed that one sentence to define me.

I wish I could've verbalized this at a younger age, but a key factor in my periods of great sadness was struggling with things that should have been easy. Some things that others thought difficult were easy for me, but routine things that people take for granted can seem impossible. This is what made the racing families I had at SKUSA and USAC so amazing; they accepted that some things were difficult for me. But here were people at an organization serving the autism community who *did not* understand. With one sentence from that woman, I began to hate myself.

On the racing side of life, Jerry Coons Jr. became USAC's Quarter Midget director. As a driver, Jerry won USAC's Triple Crown—series championships in Silver Crown, Sprint Cars, and Midgets—and working with him was a joy. He came from a racing background, so he looked at things from a different viewpoint from his predecessors. He trusted my input regarding rules, and he brought a level of professionalism that was refreshing. However, with the trouble I was having on my primary job, I wasn't enjoying the race weekends as I had.

In my day job, I noticed a decrease in my opportunities to write as the year went along. More and more meetings were scheduled, and each meeting seemed to focus on the last meeting and the next meeting; nothing was ever really said, and nothing ever done. It was a circular pattern of nonsense that made no sense to me.

As I've said, people on the spectrum can be naïve about workplace politics. I cared about one thing only: giving as much hope as possible to anyone who heard my message. But David spent more time talking about *how* to present than talking about the actual content.

In October, I had another one of those moments that defined how I felt about myself. David called a meeting and began by talking about how the onus was on him to get me more speaking opportunities. Then I was told that through my blog and presentations, I had to justify my existence. My blog was seeing record readership. Through the blog and at presentations, I was getting praise from parents who said they finally understood their kids. If that wasn't enough justification, what would be?

For those on the spectrum, this thought—*I am not good enough*—is a pit of darkness almost impossible for the soul to escape. However, the year of pain wasn't close to being over.

As the fourth quarter began, there was a meeting with several directors. For reasons I never quite understood, this small meeting was held in an open room where a larger public meeting was about to take place. There I was told that my presentations weren't all that important and I'd have to stay in the office more. When I asked what I'd be doing, they said they didn't know; for persons on the spectrum, there's a need to know what's expected, but they couldn't tell me.

Then they said that I'd have to end my law-enforcement presentations because, "After all, Aaron, who is that actually helping?" I'd been told by officers of cases in which my words had "saved a life" because the officers either de-escalated the situation or at least did not escalate the level of force used. This was irrelevant. Those statements of those officers were forgotten, and once again I was hearing: "Not good enough."

I was also told that my blog would no longer be part of the job. "It's not like people read it," someone said. "Besides, this will make your life easier." Gaslighting at its finest.

In December, I had the honor of being invited to the FBI Behavioral Analysis Unit (BAU) conference. The BAU agents are the bureau's "profilers." They don't deal with many civilian presentations, but after I did one for the FBI's

St. Louis field office earlier in 2016, someone there thought that it was of "high importance" that I do a presentation for the BAU. It was a momentary win during a year of questioning my worth. But when I got home, David said, "Aaron, why'd you do that presentation? Who did you think it helped? There was no reason to do that. Don't waste time like that."

While spending Christmas at my mom's house in Nebraska, I realized this job was killing me. Even though my sense of self-worth was low, I knew I was above the way they were treating me. I wrote a strong email reflecting that belief, but the meetings and gaslighting continued. I was always to blame. I wasn't "innovative" enough.

In February of 2017, I'd gone to the north side of St. Louis to give a presentation. While I was waiting in the parking lot, I wrote an email saying that if this was a "constructive dismissal," I would put in my two-week notice. As with the time I sent a girlfriend a Christmas breakup text just to see if she still liked me, I somehow expected that this email would put things right. And much like in that old breakup, I was wrong. During my presentation, I got an email back. That was that. A job that had meant so much to me was gone. My title, which had served so well as the "alias" under which I could function, was gone, too. And I felt like I, as a human, was gone as well, unable to be saved, and worthy of nothing.

—— Racing On My Own in 2017 ——

NOT TOO LONG AFTER THE LOSS OF MY JOB, I BECAME A business owner and began making presentations on my own. Eventually I would get an agent, but to start with, 2017 saw lots of amazing venues but not much revenue. Over the course of the year, I presented at several FBI functions in California, and I also became a presenter at the FBI National Academy, said to be one of the hardest institutions to be accepted into. I guess being a presenter there meant I was worthy of *something*, but I didn't see it. I was still trying to "justify my existence," and live up to a standard that was impossible to achieve.

Racing started off earlier than normal, with SKUSA starting a winter series in Florida. This helped the bank account and was a temporary reprieve from the exercise of trying to justify my existence.

I was a bitter person during this time frame, and almost every conversation with my dad would eventually spiral downward until I concluded, *again*, that, "everything is wrong because I'm not good enough." There's a reason the unemployment rate for those with Asperger's is so high and this is one of them. I was traumatized, damaged, and after an experience like that, how could I simply go back? It was that old trap: If failure is a guarantee, what's the logic in trying?

The USAC .25 Midget series opened the season in Phoenix in conjunction with IndyCar and the USAC Silver Crown series. I got to do double duty as a flagman, handling the .25 Midget action and the Silver Crown feature. Jerry Coons Jr. was also multitasking; in addition to serving as director of the .25 Midgets, he'd be racing in the Silver Crown event.

It was my first Silver Crown race as chief starter, and also my first at the legendary Phoenix International Raceway. Walking from the Quarter Midget track over to the big track brought a smile to my face, and smiles were in short supply for me then. As I climbed into the flagstand and looked over the Phoenix mile, I felt a flood of relief. It was a huge honor to be given this job.

This was also neat for me because I was once again flagging in front of IndyCar. The Silver Crown feature was on Saturday afternoon, with the IndyCar race that evening. During our pre-race activities, I nodded at Jim Swintal, who had been the chief starter for Championship Auto Racing Teams (CART) and was now the voice of race control for IndyCar. He probably had no idea who I was, but he nodded back. Once again, I smiled.

I turned and started putting the flags in the holder and … I was short one flag! Somehow, I didn't have a white flag with me. In a panic I called Steve, the Quarter Midget race director, and there was no answer. I left a voicemail and a text message, hoping he could run my primary white flag over to me. Meanwhile, I thought of ways to mimic a white flag in case that was necessary. We were just a couple minutes from engines firing, so I looked at the stands below and saw a fan who had several white towels. I hurried down the ladder and explained my problem, and he happily lent me a white flag … uh, towel.

As the engines started, I saw Steve walking toward me on the concourse, smiling at my problem but holding my white flag. I said, "You might as well stay," so he was my backup.

A Silver Crown race on a paved oval is an experience. In the stand, all that horsepower created a rumble that I could feel running through me. Anytime I'm flagging something new, I worry about making a mistake. I knew the rules and I knew the flags, but there's still a level of doubt until I've done something and put it behind me. But after the laps wound down and I flew the double-checkered flags over winner Bobby Santos, I had to admit that I'd had a flawless performance. I smiled as the last car went by, thinking, "Wow, what a cool job this is!"

As I descended the ladder, several people were waiting to say that they appreciated my flag-waving skills. This was something new, as were the wandering hands of two older women who'd had a bit too much to drink and seemed to like the flagmen!

A couple of months later, the USAC .25 Midgets had a three-night event at Tri-City Speedway in Granite City, Illinois, just across the Mississippi River from St. Louis. I hadn't done anything with the local kart club for eight years, so it felt good to have a home race.

We'd now had a few races with Jerry at the helm of the series, and as a group we were starting to gel. No matter what I'm doing, I've always struggled with staff turnover. I'm not one to say "this is how Kyle did it" or "that's the way it's always been," but with a new person comes a new routine, and that means change.

This was the first USAC race my then-girlfriend would get to watch. She had heard the stories of my broken bones and ambulance rides, so I convinced her to come to see how safe it is.

Halfway through the second day, she was walking toward the grid area, and I saw the announcer talking to her. I thought this odd, because she really didn't know anyone at the track, but I could see that she had a look of dismay on her face. After the next race finished and I had some time, I turned to her and asked, "Something wrong?"

There was no immediate answer. What could the announcer possibly have told her that would impact me? Was I about to be fired?

Another race came and went, and after the checkered flag I turned to her again and said, "Seriously, what's wrong?" Was she about to break up with me?

She didn't speak, and another race rolled out. This one went quickly, green to checkered with no yellows. I got out of the stand and said, "Tell me!"

"I can't," she replied, looking at the ground. "It will destroy you."

Destroy? I began to panic. What news would destroy me? "Please," I said. "Tell me."

She looked up into my eyes and said, "It's Kyle. He's gone. He drowned."

Grief

"AARON … AARON…" MY GIRLFRIEND KEPT SAYING. "AARON, it was a boating accident." She gave me the facts, but I couldn't comprehend. It was sudden. It was unexpected. It was the end. How? Why? I couldn't make sense of it. She was right, it destroyed me.

The next race had pushed out of the pits, and the sound of engines broke the silence in my head. Instead of getting into the flagstand, I got out my phone. I went to Facebook Messenger and opened up the chat with Kyle. It read: "Last active 8 hours ago." Surely this bad news was a mistake. We'd just communicated eight hours ago. This couldn't be reality. Things like this happen on the news, not to someone I would know. I never had lost a friend, and I was frozen.

As the cars circled, and the drivers slotted into their assigned starting positions, I looked up. My coworkers could tell I had received the news, and no one wanted to radio me to take my position. With tears flowing, I took the stand and flagged on for the rest of the day.

Again, there's that misconception about people on the autism spectrum: that they don't have emotions towards others or may just use others to get what they want. I hate hearing those kinds of generalizations, and I hate to hear stories from those on the spectrum who've been told those things when they *know* otherwise. That stuff is not the truth. We just have such a difficult time socializing in the traditional way.

But Kyle … in the thousands of miles we drove together, he got to see the real me, something only a few have been able to achieve.

To get to know me well, a person would have to work with me directly and make small talk, mixed in with doing the actual job or traveling to the job. Much like a tornado, the elements must be just right. Otherwise, I'll remain my closed self. And Kyle was now … gone.

When the day's races were finished, I drove home in a mental fog. Kyle had been trying to call me for about a month, but because I was getting more and more depressed about my job being gone, I wasn't up to hearing him being his usual cheerful self.

I once again opened up Messenger and saw our last conversation:

Kyle: "Liketens, why you ignore all my calls?"

Me: "You keep calling when I can't talk, or am not awake."

Kyle: "You read my text and still didn't call."

Knowing he had me, I responded with a simple, "Can't talk now."

Kyle, with his spot-on way of knowing when things stank said, "What? You in a library all day?"

I sat on this for a day, and responded, "Life sucks, and I'm not in much of a talking mood. I need a miracle."

His last message to me was, "Well you can't get ideas if you don't talk to people."

Those last words were haunting. He had mentioned many times to me that I wasn't *that* different from everyone. In a previous conversation, when we discussed the worsening situation at my job, he said he understood what "constructive dismissal" was and could relate to my words. As I write this, thinking about the day after we heard the news and the somber tone at the track—by now, everyone knew, and a moment of silence had been observed—it felt like I had lost a family member. I could never have prepared for the sense of loss I experienced losing a brother-by-work-place. Even more so, I couldn't imagine the grief his actual family was experiencing.

In the following days, details on the services were announced. I knew I couldn't go. How could I? Sure, by not going I was playing into the misconception that Aspies are uncaring jerks, but going, to use my girlfriend's term, would have *actually* destroyed me. So, I did what I do when I can't express myself with spoken words: I wrote. I posted the following on Facebook:

"I don't know what's supposed to be said at a funeral. Truth is, I've only been to one and I didn't really know the person. That said, again, I don't know what's supposed to be said and I know I would never be able to verbalize these words, so I'll do what a writer does and write...

"Kyle ... there's no single word that comes to mind when trying to describe him and I think that's the definition of a person that truly lived. I had the pleasure of working with him at the USAC .25 series for six years and traveled coast to coast several times and in those times everyday events became stories. Stories though doesn't quite sound right because when Kyle would tell a story it wasn't just an everyday occurrence, but he could make the mundane sound extraordinary and the extraordinary sound, well, even extraordinarier. Did you hear him tell the story of the one restaurant that messed his order up four times? Or how about the time he convinced a federal park ranger that he didn't have the keys for the trailer he was pulling because he had, well, let's say the right permits weren't in hand. If you didn't hear those stories, try and imagine how well he'd tell it and multiply it tenfold. And of course, I'm sure you heard about the story of the time a Quarter Midget landed on him.

"It didn't matter if it was about the race we just worked or the Bengals' dismal playoff hopes, he spoke every word with a zest I envied. He found humor at times others couldn't and came up with one-liners that would live on for many years thereafter. And speaking of those one-liners, he would know they were awesome and when those around him would be cracking up he'd deadpan it and say 'What?'

"At my final race I worked with him at the conclusion of the 2015 season in Lansing, the staff had a dinner at a restaurant right by the track and I'll admit I cried that day because

I feared what was to come. I'd grown so accustomed to his mannerisms, and rooming with him for so long that I knew of the 40-minute showers in the morning, that it was like losing ... a friend. I keep to myself normally and it's part by choice, part because I'm on the autism spectrum. Through the years he learned, accepted, and accommodated my challenges. When I'm uncomfortable I'll typically struggle in silence and at the next-to-last race we worked, we went into a restaurant that had live drums being played. I have severe sensory issues to those, and I didn't need to say a word. He told the others, 'Nope, this isn't going to work,' and we went elsewhere. This wasn't the move of a coworker but of a true friend, which is why that final meal I had was difficult ... because I knew the way I am and that I would not reach out to say hello, or to try and get a round of hilarious golf in.

"I started by saying he truly lived, but I know a character like he was lived more than most ever will. He traveled more miles than most, cared more than most despite trying not to show it, and certainly worked harder than most people I've met. And of course, told more stories and had more ideas (with a raised finger, of course) than any 10 people combined. That said, I know he will live on in us all because there's no forgetting a person like that. I mean, did he tell you about the time that one professional player blocked him on Twitter? Or that he gave a certain NASCAR driver his nickname? He was larger than life, and his memory and stories for all who knew him will be remembered for all time."

The pastor ended the funeral service with what I wrote, and I was told he did a great job. But I was still angry at myself for not having the strength to go.

Maybe I got lucky. Maybe this level of grief is experienced by others earlier in life. I wish the misconceptions were true: I wish I *didn't* care. I wish I could tell you with a straight face that I'm immune to emotions, because when those emotions hit, they consume me.

When Right is Right in the Midst of Confusion

THE FOLLOWING MONTHS REMAIN A BLUR. MY ANGER AT losing my job embittered my soul. Sure, I had my presentations, and at some extraordinary venues, but the loss of my title and now being an independent business owner clouded my ability to see who I really was.

Oh, and I was still fixated on those four heart-piercing words: "It's not that difficult." Because it *was* that difficult, even in racing, which had always been a respite for me. At the 2017 SKUSA SuperNationals, I was put in the uncomfortable position of either doing what I knew to be wrong or speaking up to question authority.

It was Friday, the longest day of the SuperNats because it's the day practice and qualifying give way to wheel-to-wheel competition. It may be the longest, but it's my favorite day for that very reason.

Early in a race in the master's category, there was a crash that blew open a big hole in the Tecpro barriers. The repair would take too long to complete safely under green-flag conditions, so a full-course yellow was called.

Prior to this event, I filmed a flag-explanation video so drivers would know what was expected of them when various flags were used. For example, full-course yellows aren't common in karting, especially for those traveling from Europe, so I gave a detailed explanation on the usage of two yellows, and that when we were ready to go back to racing, I'd show the field a rolled-up green flag to indicate the race would resume next time by.

The incident scene had been cleared, and the track was almost repaired. I radioed to control, "Control, are we go for one-to-green next time by?" There was no answer. The field was three turns from the straight and I radioed again,

"Control, recommending one-to-green?" The person working as control responded, "Go green!"

"Say again?" I responded. I heard, but I couldn't do it. The field was strung out a bit, as I'd instructed them to be in the video, and again at the driver's meeting. I couldn't throw the green flag with no one expecting it. Or could I? I had shades of Modesto 2014, when we walked on each other's transmissions, and the time I questioned the race director in front of the drivers, which earned me a tongue lashing.

Control shouted, "Throw the damn green!" The leader was already at my feet, so I didn't. Not that I would've. I radioed, "We *must* give a one to green signal. We must!" Control was in turn four and as the field got there, they gave the "let loose" hand signal. Confusion reigned.

I radioed, "We are not green. The green was not displayed at the finish line. The track is still full-course yellow."

Control retorted, "Drop your yellows! Why aren't we green? Why do the corner workers have the yellows displayed?"

This was now a situation where all control had been lost. Half the corner workers listened to me, and the other half listened to her. The drivers were also confused. Some maintained the pace of a full-course yellow while others saw this as a chance to greatly improve their positions. I remained at the line with two yellow flags displayed, the indication of a full-course yellow.

If I could've frozen time, I would've. We needed to get on the same page because a dangerous situation was brewing. Could I just "let go" and allow the person working as control to fall on her own sword? It was her mistake, but at the same time, would it be fair to those who traveled thousands of miles to be screwed by a misunderstanding of the restart procedure? I told myself after being yelled at by a race director years ago that I'd always do exactly as I was told, but this wasn't right. Starts and restarts were my department; my face was literally on the video that acted as an extension of the rulebook. If what I was doing was wrong, I'd take the blame. But this time I was more than right and this, for me, was a battle worth fighting for.

The karts were now coming onto the main straight, and I maintained my double yellow. The drivers knew something was up, so the karts that had been at full speed suddenly slowed down and the karts behind them veered, slid, and almost spun at this unexpected slowdown. Control came on the radio, "Aaron, this is on you! You want to kill someone? Do you even know what's going on right now?" I wanted to respond that they were the ones lost.

There was just one thing to do as we were burning laps and that was to trust the drivers to get in the right position, so as the leaders approached, I got out the green and, as I assured all the drivers I would do, I showed the one-to-green signal.

You can't always trust drivers to do the right thing. So often the saying is, "the helmet goes on and the brain turns off." However, what happened next shocked me; these drivers were signaling each other, even surrendering positions they'd gained during our lap of confusion.

That entire lap, race control was yelling at me on the radio, but I was at the point where I didn't care. This person didn't know the restart procedure, and right was truly right, and we were going to restart the race next time by.

The field made their way around the lap in an orderly fashion. It was time once again for my "playing in traffic" restart. I held my breath as I looked up the long straight to see the leader, and 30 plus other drivers wanting his position.

Slowly they made their way to me. Control was still barking at me, but I was tuned out unless I heard the word, "Abort!" which would mean to wave the yellow. Other than that, I was not listening. I had lost faith in what they knew. When the lead kart reached the restart zone, it accelerated and I flew the green high, then I began to run and finally jumped over the barrier— "the Likens leap," Rob Howden called it—as the race resumed.

The adrenaline now hit me. This was a high-intensity moment; I'd done something I told myself I'd never do again. I'd gone against authority. The personal attacks I endured on the radio now had gotten to me.

Aside from occasional tiffs with competitors when I'd been a race director, it had been a long time since I was spoken to like this. Sure, there'd been the odd heckling spectator, and the sarcastic standing ovation I got when I freed my yellow flag from the catch fence at Columbus Motor Speedway just in time to give a one-to-green. But this was personal, and uncalled for.

Conflict resolution isn't an Aspie's strong suit, and I shut down. I continued to do my job with the same care as I always had, but I could no longer speak. There was no advocating to the race director, only silence. To confirm halfway and two-to-go, I gave hand signals to scoring; Tony Leone later told me that the scorers kept saying, "It wasn't us," wanting me to know that they were not part of this issue. But while a tempest swirled inside me, the quality of work didn't diminish.

That night the race director did ask for my input on what happened in that race, because some drivers were angry about having lost positions under yellow-flag conditions. After my explanation, he understood, and the next day the person working control apologized to me; she hadn't understood the difference between the practice procedure, where after a full-course yellow we'd just go green, and race procedure, in which restart rules needed to be followed. I was assured the mistake would not happen again, and it never has.

Looking back on that night, it could've played out much worse. With the level of depression I had after the loss of

Kyle and the loss of my job, I could've just said, "I'm done!"

But that would have meant walking away from the sport I love.

Flagging with Mario

WITH 2018 CAME NEW SPEAKING VENUES, AND MANY MORE opportunities to speak at various FBI conferences and field offices. I worked with an FBI Victim Specialist in Ohio, and helped a person on the spectrum understand the emotions they had and offered advice should they decide to become a public speaker. Things were … well, they were good, but I was still trapped in feeling "not good enough."

Reading this, you may be yelling at me out loud for not being able to see the blessings right in front of me. But this is a pitfall of life on the autism spectrum. I wanted to be happy; I didn't want to feel only despair. But I finally let a workplace become family, and then people in that "family" questioned my every move and said my work was "not good enough."

On the racing side, it was going to be a busy year with USAC and SKUSA. I was now going to travel to California six times to work the SKUSA Pro Kart Challenge, which is their regional series out there. This worked out great because I also became affiliated, as a contractor, to present for Easterseals Southern California.

For the 2018 USAC .25 Midget season, a new series director took over for Jerry Coons Jr., with Danielle Frye taking the helm. Danielle came from an extensive background in NASCAR, having been a pit reporter for MRN radio and also having served as senior manager of communications for the sanctioning body. All of the directors before Danielle were professional, but, with her connections, she brought things to a whole new level.

The 2018 calendar saw us running at tracks where NASCAR or IndyCar were running, so we'd be set up as a sideshow of sorts to gain the attention of passing fans, who would stop to watch and turn us into a real attraction. Beyond that, Danielle had a habit of securing some amazing honorary starters. At Phoenix, we had the legendary Mario Andretti.

IndyCar was racing the one-mile oval, and I was giddy to pull double duty once more by flagging the returning USAC Silver Crown Series. But what I wondered most was whether Mario would be just making an appearance at the Quarter Midget track, or if he'd wave a green flag on one of our races.

I'm not sure our young drivers truly appreciated who Mario is, and what he has achieved in his brilliant career. But if they hadn't, their parents must have filled them in, because when Mario arrived at the Quarter Midget track, he was essentially mobbed by the young racers. They almost knocked him down. He was gracious, polite, and always smiled. I was astounded at the composure he had and the grace with which he spoke with the kids.

Opening ceremonies came and went and the rookie class took to the track, with Mario still in the pit area. It wouldn't be the end of the world if he didn't come over to wave the green. In fact, I worried a bit about what might happen if he did. I'd recently had a few more Quarter Midgets strike my flagstand injuring me; I think I was averaging one hospital visit per season for racing crashes in which I wasn't a driver, and I'd hate to see anything happen to someone else, especially someone like Mario.

And then, there he was. Danielle walked over with Mario, and as they arrived, she whispered to me, "You're welcome." I was about to have Mario Andretti as an honorary starter. It gave me chills then, and it gives me chills now, writing this.

I was introduced to Mario, as if he needed any introduction at all. Before the next heat rolled out, we talked about the kids, the schedule, the places we go, and he was intensely focused on my words. He truly wanted to know where these kids raced, and what the next potential step would be for them.

He didn't need much briefing, but I asked, "Do you need any kind of prompt when the race begins?" He smiled, shook his head, and the kids in that heat took the green from Mario.

As the laps went by, he stayed beside me. A yellow flag came out, and during this caution period he made observations about some of the drivers in the middle of the pack. He had his eye on one in particular; she was running a different line that he liked. Then Mario asked if he could wave the green for the restart. There was zero chance of him getting a "no" answer from me.

I gave the one-to-go signal, handed Mario the green, and again his flagging skills were spot on. He even added a bit of style. In the grand scheme of things, that day at Phoenix won't make even a blip on his list of accomplishments, but you should know that the man can flag!

With the laps ticking down, he and I began commentating on the race we were watching. The driver he'd mentioned earlier was making moves. We talked over the engines about the different apexes, the passes, the crossover passes. It went by all too fast, as I handed him the white flag and then the checkered flag. There's a picture out there of me looking over his shoulder with the biggest smile on my face; he's leaning over the barriers with the same look of focus I'd have expected to have seen at Monaco in 1978.

When the cars pulled off, I shook his hand, and he thanked me. As he departed, I said, "If I need a break, I know who to call. You were amazing at this!" He was, and one thing I learned that day—and it's a credo I've tried to live by since then: You can't fake passion.

Yes, no matter how good a person might be at something, if there's no passion involved, the work will show it. Mario's passion for motorsports oozed from him. He could've "phoned in" this detour to the Quarter Midget track by waving the green and hurrying back to the IndyCar paddock, but he took the time to learn about the cars and the kids, and even worked as the flagger for one race.

For those on the spectrum, when I talk about employment, I say again: You can't fake passion. We often will attempt to find a job in an interest we love dearly, and when we do, that passion we have will shine through. I saw what lasting passion looks like when talking with Mario Andretti, and I can only hope that at some point, someone looks at me and sees passion there, whether I'm waving flags at a race track or making a presentation on behalf of those on the autism spectrum.

2019: A Year of Close Calls

MAY OF 2019 ROLLED AROUND, AND I WAS STILL IN A SLOW bleed of sadness. I was making presentations, but the financial blow of losing a full-time job was creating an almost unbearable amount of anxiety for me. Waking up in the morning, I felt like I had a ton of bricks sitting on my chest. The words "not good enough" went through my head each hour. I began to wonder if maybe the website I'd read long ago, on the night of my diagnosis, was accurate after all. However, with the month of May came my favorite traditions of the year, my favorite races, and perhaps a respite from the drama of life.

I had worked the Hoosier Hundred with Tom Hansing for many years, but this year a person I didn't know, Erik, would be the main starter, with me as the assistant. We split qualifying and he had me flag the UMP Modified feature, which was an amazing race. As the pre-Hoosier Hundred ceremonies began, things like finances, job loss, and the future didn't register in my brain. I was … *happy*!

Making the night even more special was that, along with my dad, I had a friend in from Canada. They were seated just five or six rows behind me, and it felt like a treat having family and friends so close.

The USAC Silver Crown series had a bit of a resurgence going, and a great field of cars turned up at the Indiana State Fairgrounds. The three-wide start at the Indy 500 will always be my favorite sight at any race track, but seeing 32 Silver Crown cars rolling out of turn four on a perfect evening, just as the sun has gone down, is also high on the list. The thing that set the Indianapolis Fairgrounds apart, in terms of the flagstand, was that we were using a platform that extended off the front row seats of the grandstands. Our feet were just above the top of the roll cages on the cars, and this provided a sensory experience I haven't felt anywhere else. I'm sure I felt my internal organs move around a couple inches as the race began, and the pack dove into turn one.

The trouble spots I helped Erik watch for were the entry to turn one and the hard-to-see turn three. This was my tenth Hoosier Hundred, and history had shown the entry to the corners were the trouble spots.

With five laps complete, thing started settling into a nice rhythm. A 100-mile Silver Crown event has an endurance-race feel; those who lead early might not lead later, because a driver has to balance running hard and fast with saving tires for the end. Tire failures often happen late in these races, but on this night, lap six saw one of the scariest blowout crashes ever.

I was looking towards turn four as the leaders came off the corner. My eyes were drawn to Chris Windom, the early leader. As he got halfway between turn four and our location, it looked like his right rear tire expanded in a way I couldn't comprehend and then collapsed in on itself. The tire had shredded, and now Windom was just a passenger as the car veered hard into the wall. After contact, the car launched into the air, and life started going frame-by-frame. That 1,625-pound car looked like a toy as it bounced and flew. I questioned the physics in play; it all looked impossible. The car started rolling in the air, and I then noticed I was looking up as it soared closer. Many thoughts occurred all at once. The first was for my father, seated behind me: Great, my dad is going to see me as a pancake.

The fence at the Indy mile left a lot to be desired. If this car got into it, Erik and I would likely be in serious trouble.

I know I screamed and scrunched down in a brace position. The next emotion I felt was regret. Had I squandered my life? When you think you're about to get squashed by a race car in flight, it's easy to forget about the *good* things. As full of regret and remorse as I was at times, there had also been some highlights. I had spoken to over 90,000 people!

Now I heard the loudest crashing noise of my life.

I opened my eyes, and Chris's car was maybe five feet from my face. But it was five feet *past* me. I knew then that I'd be okay, although the car was still tumbling violently. Erik had dived down, so there was *no* flag being displayed. Without thought, on instinct alone, I grabbed the red flag and started waving furiously. I do remember not looking towards turn one, because I didn't want to see the result if Windom's car was struck by another at 150 miles per hour. The sound of that secondary collision never came. All the cars somehow avoided the crashed car, which settled in a bent heap. It was soon apparent that Chris was okay, even if shaken up a bit. A radio call came from the race director asking if we were okay in the flagstand. Erik looked at me, I looked at him, and we both nodded, knowing that we were lucky to still be experiencing life on this Earth. I think we both would've been okay if the race ended there.

During the cleanup of the crash, I sat by my dad and stared off in silence.

Close calls and impacts from Quarter Midgets were something I'd become all too familiar with. But had this crash tossed Windom's car differently, by just a few degrees, my story might have ended that night. Erik knew this feeling, too.

When the race was restarted, it all felt different, as if we were tempting fate. Drivers willingly take the risks and look danger square in the eyes every time they take the wheel, and those that work at the races do, also. But when something like this happens, it's hard to once again let go of control and play the odds.

The checkered flags flew at the end of the race; Tyler Courtney won, but I don't remember that unless I look it up. I don't remember turning in my radio or leaving the track. I do remember that when we got to Kimberly's condo, I told my dad, "I'm done. I can't do this anymore."

I was scheduled to assist at the next evening's Carb Night Classic at Indianapolis Raceway Park, but I called and said I couldn't. The person I talked to knew why. It didn't have to be spoken. The Windom crash had shaken a lot of people. This would be the first event I signed up for, but then didn't do. And it wasn't the only event I thought about skipping.

Perhaps that crash triggered something along the lines of a midlife crisis, but I looked at my personal history to that point. Again, I'd had my share of emergency-room visits, and in addition to some of the injures I've already mentioned, I had micro-fractures to my femur, I'd broken my tailbone twice, I'd endured several sprained ankles, and picked up enough bruises to last a lifetime. Did I need this? Maybe my mom was right, maybe I needed to stop playing in traffic. Perhaps the level of danger had exceeded my passion for the sport. Besides, if I never made it to the top, would all these injuries have been worth it?

The first mistake in my reasoning was judging everything against whether I made it to the top. To have an impossible goal and to set that as your bar of success is not good, because it diminishes all the other good things you may do. I really did love every race I worked, and I was good at what I did. So, I had not been a failure.

Then, at right around the time someone else was waving the green flag at Indianapolis Raceway Park, I came across a photo on Facebook. I mentioned that the night before, on instinct alone, I had grabbed the red flag and waved it. I didn't remember this. But someone had posted a photo of the Windom car in the air, one bounce after the flagstand, and clearly visible is my red flag. While I'd been feeling defeated, ready to retire, here was a photo showing that in a moment of great danger I maintained enough composure to do my job and to warn other drivers that this was a bad situation.

My desire to retire went away, but depression remained with me the rest of the year. I was close to doing enough speaking gigs to support myself, but I was still knocking at the door of being able to make a profit.

Things came to a head when I was in Las Vegas for the USAC .25 Midget event. I was in my hotel room, just thinking about things. For those of us on the autism spectrum, logic can be used for good, but when *flawed* logic enters our thoughts, it can make cloudy everything we know. The fail-set mindset had control of me again. I'd been doing my presentations at some amazing venues, yet I was allowing myself to be defined by people and events from two years earlier.

The evening before the finals in Vegas had me awake all night, crying most of the hours. I tried to write down my emotions, but what was the point? I had one line—"No one reads your stuff anyway"—reverberating through my brain.

I thought: What if there is no tomorrow? What if I'm not part of everyone else's tomorrow? Horrible thoughts. I often question whether I write too much about my dark days, but I think it's impossible for someone to find meaning in my successes if they don't understand how low I had gotten. And there I was in Las Vegas, at maybe the lowest low.

Taking stock of my life that night, I finally saw that each dark time in my life was followed up by something amazing. So maybe it would happen again. Life may have been bleak for me, and I didn't know how I'd find my way out of the pattern I was in, but there was no reason to give up. Something was bound to happen because it always had.

Faith can be hard to find when everything appears lost. But I still had mine.

The Big One at Daytona

DANIELLE FRYE HAD CULTIVATED THE RELATIONSHIP between USAC and NASCAR, and our first race of 2020 was at the Daytona International Speedway on the weekend of NASCAR's Busch Clash and ARCA 200 weekend. This was great, because it started my season earlier, and because it was a neat sensation to be flagging Quarter Midgets in an infield parking lot and be able to look up and see stock cars practicing on the banking.

There was a bit of apprehension as we got to Daytona, as more and more news reports were saying something about a coronavirus, the newly named COVID-19. At the time though, this was a problem mostly limited to China and beginning to appear in Italy. In the U.S., it wasn't yet something that seemed imminently dangerous.

The USAC .25 Midget event at Daytona was so popular they had to limit the number of entries. This may have been a "youth series," but the competition was far fiercer than when I'd started with the group 10 seasons earlier.

On the third day of the event, it was cold for Florida. The clear skies and bright sun hid the fact that jackets were required. About an hour before we were to begin racing, someone gave me some Crunch 'n Munch popcorn. Ah, they didn't know the curse. Crunch 'n Munch may taste amazing, but each time I'd been given Crunch 'n Munch on the morning of a race, I'd ended up in the hospital. I'm not superstitious, but the facts showed that having this food at a race was tempting fate. I told the person who gave it to me, "You have no idea what you've just done."

It was in the first handful of races that morning that it happened. One car lost a chain and began to slow. I waved the yellow flag and most everyone eased up, but the kid in last place came around turns three and four at full speed. I could actually look into the helmet of that kid and see where he was looking; he was looking at his own front bumper, rather than ahead. By the time he saw that the other cars had slowed for a yellow flag, it was too late. He veered at the last possible moment, but still hit the right-rear tire of the kid in front.

When open-wheel cars touch tires, it's not uncommon for the trailing car to get airborne as his tires climb the tires of the car ahead. Sure enough, the Quarter Midget of the kid who hadn't been looking far enough ahead jumped into the air and angled right, heading for the wall in front of me. With the angle, speed, and height he had, he got over that wall and made direct contact with my small flagstand. The impact was brutal, and I was flung forward into the railing of the stand. The stand rotated, and, as a witness to the crash said, "Aaron's body twisted all sorts of wrong ways."

I was whipped forward, then back, with an awful twisting motion at my torso.

When the crashing stopped, I attempted to stand. I saw medics running my way, and they were motioning for me to get back down. Having just realized that the wind had been literally knocked out of me, "back down" was exactly the position I went to.

In some of my other incidents where injuries occurred, there had been discussions about whether a hospital visit was in order. At Daytona, they didn't give me a choice. I was loaded into the ambulance and driven to Halifax Medical Center.

It was now official: The Crunch 'n Munch curse had struck again.

I made sure to say that the only pain I had was in my knees and torso. My neck was fine, and I didn't want to spend a couple hours on a backboard with my head strapped down, but the medics that witnessed the crash weren't taking chances.

In the emergency room, the first thing I heard a nurse say was, "A person from the track? I didn't think ARCA was running until tomorrow!" It was difficult to explain that I wasn't a driver; I'd been hit by a car. No, not a passenger car, as you'd first think when someone says "hit by a car," but a little race car that obviously packed a big punch.

The usual X-rays and tests were taken. Outside of bruising, I appeared fine, so I was released after a few hours. Two days later, after landing in Indianapolis to drive home to St. Louis, I noticed a big bulge by my navel; had I been more injured than I suspected? I visited my doctor in St. Louis, who said I had a traumatic abdominal wall hernia, and surgery was required.

My concern was whether I'd have time to recover before the SKUSA WinterNationals in New Orleans. The gap was 10 days. I had the surgery, a doctor signed off that I was okay to travel, and I flew to New Orleans in time for the weekend when everything changed.

The End of the World as I Knew It

As I got to the airport to fly to Louisiana, there was an abundance of people wearing masks. It was March 11, 2020, and there was a viral storm coming. It hadn't hit yet, but it was obvious that *something* was about to happen. How bad would it be? I remembered previous viral scares, and none of them had made a major national impact. But during our first practice in New Orleans, we learned that an NBA basketball game was postponed due to a COVID infection. The talk now picked up; it was clear that everyday life could be impacted. As the day progressed, I started getting texts from people about events possibly being postponed or cancelled.

On Friday, COVID was the only thing discussed. When practice began, I could tell that my body wasn't fully ready for a weekend of racing. In the second session, a kart caught one of our communication wires and brought it onto the track. This required quick action, so I ran to clear the debris. Right away, my body told me that running was a bad idea. Much like the night of the previous year's Hoosier Hundred, I questioned if this was the best thing I could be doing with my life. Maybe I had been hurt too many times.

Before lunch, I got a text from a friend working the IndyCar opener in St. Petersburg. Because of the COVID situation, they were on standby; they eventually postponed. Then we heard that NASCAR was going to postpone its

Homestead race. As we completed a round of practice in New Orleans, we were told there would be a "break." This break wasn't planned, and I figured it could mean only one thing.

The world was shutting down, and so, too, was our SKUSA event. "Get home" was the message. The world was changing by the minute, to a degree few of us had ever seen. SKUSA was gracious enough to still pay us and get us on flights early the next day.

At the airport I talked with Preston Buckley, my assistant starter in SKUSA and USAC, about what the future might look like. Like many people, I was facing the loss of my entire revenue stream; there were no races to flag, and certainly no public-speaking opportunities. Preston thought it would be a great time to get back into iRacing. I perked up at this, and when I got back home, I signed up and even bought a new computer. If the world was going to end, I was at least going to enjoy the last days with a new computer.

Preston and I spent hours every day racing each other, and the world, on iRacing. He has the same passion for racing that I do, so it was great sharing the isolation at home with someone by chatting every day. USAC hired the two of us to direct its virtual races, which brought in some income. Kyle Larson wasn't too keen on our officiating, and tweeted, "Thought I signed up for a USAC sim race. Not a USAC Quarter Midget race with a judges table." I don't *think* he knew that actual Quarter Midget officials were behind it. He wasn't back for week two.

As the month of May began, there was little hope that the "Greatest Spectacle in Racing" would run. The reality was that the Indy 500, and most everything else, was off the table for the foreseeable future. I tried to take life one day at a time, but a tradition I'd had for decades, May in Indianapolis, was over. Of course, health and safety took precedence, but how long would this last? I did work as a commentator for iRacing's virtual Indianapolis 500. Because there were no real races, Rob Howden started commentating on iRacing events, and I lived out a bit of a dream by calling a race with him. I think I surprised him, because he said that with my skill at keeping up with race strategies, he wanted me as his spotter when he did the real-life Indianapolis 500 for the IMS Radio Network, whenever that might be.

It was also in May that the bulge returned to my navel, and it hurt like hell. The surgery had failed, and I needed another one, but the COVID situation limited the surgeries hospitals would schedule for fear of overcrowding. After a few weeks, I was finally able to make a date for the procedure.

The surgery date came, and depression had fully set in again. It's a delicate thing to write about, because I was most certainly glad I had my health, generally speaking, and I had not been physically impacted by COVID as so many had. But the emotional toll was high, and having a second surgery truly made me question, again, whether racing was something I wanted to be part of. As the anesthesia set in and things turned black, I thought: Yes, this is it. I don't need this. My racing career is over."

Coming out of anesthesia is much like picking up a television show in the middle. I was conversing before I was conscious, and as I regained control and memory, I was slamming my head on the gurney, yelling, "I wish I had never been born!" I don't know what conversations took place in my head to make me shout those words, but waking up to them was enough for me to decide that I didn't want to do anything that might lead to another surgery.

The ride home with my dad was filled with sadness. I told him, "I'm done. I'm retiring from racing. I've achieved all I can, so why should I go forward?" He didn't respond. Racing had been our thing for my entire life, and now I was disavowing my involvement in it. He knew the joy it brought me. He knew that when I'm working at a track, racing is one of the few things that keeps my brain from overthinking the stressors of life. I think it was because of this that my dad didn't respond. He wasn't going to give a verbal acceptance of my resignation from the activity I loved above all others.

Remember me saying that every time I wanted to give up, something wonderful would happen if I just hung in there? Despite being so sure that I was done with it, the racing Gods felt otherwise. They were about to open a door that had been waiting for me from the day Duane Sweeney gave me that checkered flag.

The Opening

WITHOUT HAVING TO GET READY FOR A RACE, I TOOK MY time recovering from surgery. I became dormant. What was the point of putting in any effort? It seemed the world was closed, I had no races to do, and the concept of public speaking seemed obsolete. I did have one thing to look forward to: In June, the NTT IndyCar Series would open its season at Texas Motor Speedway and that would bring a few hours of normalcy, with racing again on television.

This would be the first race I watched since my "retirement." Of course, only my dad knew what my intentions were, but I was at peace with things. Okay, so during the Texas race I might've wondered if I still had a chance to make it to that level of racing, but each time I moved in my chair brought aches and pains, reminders that my body might not want to endure more.

Several days later, though, came interesting news. *Very* interesting news. The IndyCar Series had a job opening;

they needed a chief starter. *IndyCar needed a starter.*

Could I apply? How would I apply if I did? Wait, wasn't I all done, retired?

I wrote a message to Jay Frye, president of IndyCar and the husband of Danielle Frye, the USAC .25 director. I had met Jay once, under strange circumstances. It was at the Circuit of the Americas in Austin, Texas, when the Quarter Midgets competed on an IndyCar weekend. Jay, USAC's Jason Smith, and I had an interesting discussion after one of our races that had had a confusing finish. Some of our events had a maximum-time limit, meaning that even if the full number of laps had not been completed, the race was over. This race had "timed out," and drivers were told via the one-way radio system that the race was over, and to pit. Everyone stayed on the track and completed that lap except the fourth-place driver, who pitted. Here was the quandary: The top-four finishers in that race would advance to the next round. How do you tell the driver who pitted out of fourth that he didn't advance, even though he followed the race director's instruction? Or how do you tell the driver who remained on track and thus moved up from fifth to fourth that he didn't make it? I suggested that we advance the top five, including the car that pitted; we had some leeway to do something like this in extreme circumstances, and that's what we did.

So, Jay knew who I was, and when I reached out, I quickly got a message back asking me to prepare and submit a resume. It had been a decade since I'd done anything with a resume, and I'd never prepared one for racing. I reached out to my dad and sister, Kimberly, who were extremely helpful, and my sister had the idea of including links to some videos of my flagging work. With the resume done within 24 hours, I waited.

At the same time, unbeknownst to me, a small army of people were also calling IndyCar on my behalf, recommending me as the next starter. In a time when I really needed support, I got it from a great many people I'd worked with over the years. They didn't know I needed help, and I didn't know they were helping. I may have been a poor self-promoter, but people spoke up for me without any indication that I even wanted the job. As I learned from Mario Andretti, you can't fake passion, and others will pick up on your passion. People seemed to know how much a job like this would mean to me, all based on the passion they saw.

I played the waiting game, unaware of this army in the background.

A few days later I got a call from Jon Koskey, IndyCar's senior director of technology, whose department includes race starters. This was an informal telephone interview, but an interview, nonetheless. Jon laid out the responsibilities that went with the job, including helping with what was termed "setup and teardown." For a Sunday race, we would likely get to the track the previous Tuesday, and 12-hour days were not out of the question. He also mentioned coaxial cable, fiber, ohms, and other things I didn't know. I kept saying, "Whatever is required."

The next day, I had a conference call with Jon and Kyle Novak, race director of the NTT IndyCar Series. With this call the stakes had been raised. My pulse was higher than the fear I had before my first race. I knew from experience, and from listening to the stories of others, that we Aspies don't interview well, and this was an interview over the phone; as I've mentioned, I do everything I can to avoid phones. To add to my drama, this was a conference call, and I don't do well in conversations when there's more than one person.

It was difficult to not accept failure as the interview went on. Kyle asked about my experience, which I related as factually as possible. He then asked, "So, what do you think you'd be doing in the flagstand during a race?" I found this question puzzling at first, because wouldn't it be displaying flags? But I thought back to Frankie Neidenbach, and to the race directors I'd worked with, and I realized the answer was, "I would be communicating race control's thoughts on the condition of the track, and doing exactly what you want, when you want it, and how you want it." I wanted him to be sure that I knew the starter doesn't run the race. My answer seemed to satisfy him.

The conversation went on, and near the end Kyle said, "Now, I don't know how to put this, but IndyCar is televised to a passionate fan base, and style of the flagging matters a bit. Will this be a problem?"

Finally, something I had no problem answering. I said, "This won't be a problem. Just wait until you see my double-checkered."

I probably could've used a bit more humility. But Jon chimed in and said, "I've seen the videos. He's right. The fans are going to fall in love with his moves."

They thanked me for my time, we hung up, and I was left wondering how I did.

Minutes seemed like hours, hours felt like days, and days felt like decades. The wait was agonizing. Sure, you may think, what's waiting a week or so when I'd thought about this job since Duane gave me that flag in 1990? Well, it wasn't *just* the wait. It was knowing that if I didn't get this job then, would I ever? I was knocking on destiny's door … or maybe waiting for destiny to knock on mine.

Preston kept texting, looking for me to join him on iRacing, but I spent most of that week in bed. My cat kept pawing at me, looking for me to entertain her, but even she got bored.

And then, just when I was beginning to wonder if they didn't have the heart to tell me I didn't get it, I got the job.

I got the job. My dream job! It had been a full week of waiting, wondering, and being so nervous that I forgot to breathe, but the journey was complete. It was a journey of mine from the first time I stepped on that rock in my neighborhood, and the first time I handed Frankie Neidenbach a flag. This was 30 years in the making, but the passion and dedication had paid off.

Ohm My Goodness

AFTER GETTING THE JOB, I LEARNED THAT I'D BE ONE OF THREE starters. I would work every event, and the others—Tom Hansing and Bryan Howard, whom I'd met in passing when I met Duane Sweeney—would split the season. Two starters are more useful than one, and IndyCar wanted me to gain experience working with Tom and Bryan rather than being thrown to the wolves.

I had now driven to Indianapolis from St. Louis hundreds of times, but no drive ever felt like the one I was on in 2020. Had another motorist looked over into my car that day, they'd have seen the biggest of smiles as I drove east on I-70 to Indianapolis and the start of my job at the Speedway the next day. This wasn't the Indianapolis 500, which had been rescheduled for August, but the GMR Indianapolis Grand Prix held on the road course at IMS.

It was hard to sleep knowing that the next day I'd be walking into the Speedway as the next starter. I also had to consider the social side, in that I was about to have a whole team of coworkers; prior to my call with Jon, I'd never imagined that this would be a job that required socializing. This wasn't going to be just weekends in the flagstand, but 30-40 hours of setup each race, working with a team of 12 others. This aspect of the job did make me a bit nervous.

I met Jon at the IndyCar office, across the street from IMS, and he loaded me up with the apparel I'd need. It was a whirlwind of shirts, jackets, and hellos. Then I was given my official "hard card," an all-access credential to be displayed at all times at the track. It had my name, my picture, and the word "OFFICIAL" on it.

Once the clothing was settled, it was time to head across to the track. I had worked 10 USAC Battle at the Brickyards and two EV Grands Prix, but this was different. This was IndyCar, and what I'd worked for my entire life. Before the flagstand, though, it was time to meet my coworkers and get down to the basics of the job. I'd told Jon that I knew nothing about amps, ohms, fiber meters, TSBs, timelines, and some of the other technology terms, but that I was willing to learn. To start, we arrived at the timing and scoring semi-trailer.

My first impression? I couldn't believe how much work and technology went into putting on a race. I knew about transponders and the timing lines in the track, but as Jon talked about the systems used by the series, I was beyond impressed. I envisioned race tracks as being plug-and-play operations, but oh, how little I knew!

To begin, Jon had me help the people working on pit lane. I met Bill, Rob, and Devin; Devin was new, but Bill and Rob had lots of experience at this job, which would help me. Some of my coworkers were retired from their "career" jobs, so this was their hobby that came with the perks of being as close to the action as possible. I didn't oversell my ability to anyone; I said that I knew nothing, and I quickly learned *how* little when I was tasked with using an ohmmeter. The meter showed a lot of fuzzy dots that when aligned meant one thing, and when not aligned meant something else. Panic crept in. Was my dream job going to be a nightmare instead?

On pit lane, the race teams get all their data and video through boxes we deploy, all strung together by fiber and

coaxial cable. At or near the finish line—most of the time—
is the hub of all this data, the IndyCar pit cart, which we
now wheeled to its position at the yard of bricks. I'll never
forget the weather that day; the pagoda was reflecting the
sunlight in the most majestic of ways. This was supposed to
be the happiest moment of my life; I was in IndyCar gear,
setting up for an IndyCar race. But here I was, dealing with
hundreds of feet of cable.

My weakness in being an Aspie is that it's almost impossible to ask for help. In school, I either got something
instantly or struggled in silence. Right now, on pit lane, I
was struggling in silence. I worried that I'd be laughed out
of the job, forgotten about in a month's time.

My strength as an Aspie is that I've so often fought a
losing battle; I'll fight hard, despite my panic. I'm not co-
ordinated with wires, and as I started to unspool the fiber,
I ran into tangles and knots, or what *I* thought were knots.
I'd pester Bill, who never was short on amazing one-liners;
Bill would give the cable a little jiggle, and, presto, no more
knot. I'm sure my facial expression was like a fifth-century
Roman's facial expression would have been if he suddenly
saw a jet airplane take off. I'd struggle and struggle, and
Bill's solution looked so effortless.

Mercy came at lunchtime, when at least I'd have some
time away from these new things. I smiled when the lunch
choice was Mexican; I thought back to that USAC race in
Phoenix in 2011, so happy that I'd tried Mexican food that
night. I assure you, with the start I was off to, if I told these
IMS people that I didn't do Mexican food, that might have
been the end of me.

At lunch, I met the remaining members of the team, and
it was a bit hard to keep names straight. I was asked a lot of
questions, and when they revolved around what I'd done
in racing, I was confident in my answers. When it had to
do with the work we were currently doing, I clammed up.

People asked about my previous work background, and I worried about answering. I wanted to sound competent, but not like my work was overly important. Should I mention that I'd done presentations for the FBI? Or that I'd been interviewed on national television? Was that relevant? Maybe it would show that I had skills in *something*. But would it make me seem conceited? Was this what the first day of high school was like?

After lunch, I managed to get the hang of unspooling fiber and laying it down without a tangled mess and learned how to put an end on a coaxial cable. Small steps!

At the end of the day, the field ops manager, Trent, had me go with him as we started laying fiber in the paddock. Trent said that as important as the laying out of fiber was, picking it up after a race was more critical, because there's a certain way to coil it. Since we had a moment, he unwound and laid out a 250-foot length, then showed me how fast he could re-coil it. I was astounded. This didn't seem possible. He then gave me the fiber and I attempted to give it a try, but right away I got it tangled.

Trent looked at me with some concern. He showed me in slow motion something called the "monkey-clap method." I didn't understand the name, nor could I replicate the movements he was making. At this point, I uttered, "FYI, I couldn't tie my shoes until fifth grade." I could wave a flag in fifth grade, but my fine motor skills weren't all that good, and they still weren't.

I'm not sure if we ended out of mercy, or if Trent decided I was a lost cause, but at 5:00 p.m. the team said we were in a good place and that was the workday. Two more days went the very same way. Back at my sister's place, where I was staying, I broke down. Everything I'd ever been bad at was on full display, keeping me from shining at my dream job. No one had told me I'd done badly, but no one came close to saying I'd done well, either. I was also not opening up to my coworkers, and the phrase "it's not that difficult" rang in my ears. This couldn't be how it played out; the night before practice would start, I said aloud, "This isn't going to be the way my story ends."

—— The First Flag, and the Teardown ——

THE MORNING OF THE FIRST ON-TRACK ACTIVITIES, I MET Kyle Novak, the race director who'd interviewed me over the phone, and there was a sense of intimidation there; I feared messing up before I even started. Then I was introduced to Jim Swintal, a legend and the CART starter for many years. Jim said, "Aaron, I've waited for this day. I've heard about you for years. Welcome!" As part of IndyCar's race-control team, he had a hand in the process of hiring the new starter. He said that he'd taken a lot of calls when the job opened up, and that I had many advocates saying that I deserved a chance. This calmed my nerves and allowed me to stop thinking about monkey-clapping the fiber. Jim proved to be a great mentor thanks to his flagging experience, and he would be the voice I'd be hearing on the radio.

It was July 4, race day in Indianapolis, an odd phrase to say or write. The event was the GMR Grand Prix, round two of the 2020 NTT IndyCar Series, to be run without spectators at the Indianapolis Motor Speedway. This was the new normal. But for the TV audience, the racing would be the same intense, competitive, and exhilarating action IndyCar was known for.

Tom Hansing would flag the race, but for the final warmup I was at the point in the stand. Before every practice session, we display a stationary, vertical yellow flag indicating that we're five minutes or less from the green. Sharon, the scorekeeper, radioed that it was time by calling, "Starter, five minutes." I returned a "Copy, five minutes." Then, as the clock got to 10 seconds, Jim called, "Standby, starter."

Then it came: "Green flag, starter, green flag." My first green flag working for IndyCar.

When the warmup was complete, I flew the checkered flag with an ear-to-ear smile. How lucky was I? It was incalculable.

As for the race, the start was sensory heaven as the field came off turn 14 and onto the straightaway to take the green. All that power accelerating at once as the cars sped towards turn one was a sensation felt through the entire body, and it still feels that amazing to me.

The race went almost half-distance—the 36th of 80 laps—without incident. Then the bright orange car of Oliver Askew slid through the grass and made heavy contact with the outside wall. Jim came on the radio—to us, and to the team monitoring race control—and said, "Full-course yellow, full-course yellow, pits are closed, pits are closed. Pace car, your leader is…"

Tom had been prepared and threw the double yellow flags.

The last half of the race was all green, and Scott Dixon picked up the victory. As the final laps ran down, fear began to grow. In the flagstand, I felt wonderful; working with Tom felt as natural as it had 10 months earlier, when we'd worked USAC's three-night Sprint Car Smackdown at Indiana's Kokomo Speedway. But as the flags got packed up, it was time to put away all the boxes, cables, and fibers we had deployed.

I went with Trent, who again made it look so easy. When I tried to mimic his hand motions, I couldn't make a coil anything like he did. My lack of spatial relations was on prime display, and I sensed that the end of my tenure as an IndyCar starter was near.

I found some excuse to get away from Trent and was paired with Bill and Rob on pit lane and the paddock. Picking up coaxial cable was much easier; it would not be reused, so there was no need to be perfect when picking it up. That made it great for practicing my coiling techniques. Devin saw me struggling and showed me a different method for coiling; within five minutes, I had it down. As the cable started to take shape, I screamed a loud and uncharacteristic, "Yes!" Was it perfect? No. Would it do? Absolutely. The impossible was now doable. I walked over to Bill, who was about to pick up a 250-feet strand of fiber and started coiling it myself. It took three attempts, but after the third I had a somewhat decent coil of fiber.

Next time you watch an IndyCar race on TV and the broadcast switches to something else right after the winner's interview, we'll just be getting started with our teardown. It takes four to five hours to get everything packed up, and as the trailer door shut on my first race weekend, Jon Koskey asked how things had gone.

I replied, "The flagstand was amazing!"

"Great, and the other work?"

I froze for a moment, and then said the only thing I could think of: "Whatever it takes."

He must have seen the fear in my eyes. "Well," said Jon, "hopefully we can get you to the point where the other work is amazing as well."

I nodded, turned, walked to my car, and drove out of the greatest race track in the world, not knowing whether to cry or cheer.

On the Road with IndyCar

THREE DAYS LATER, WE WERE ON THE HIGHWAY, HEADED for Wisconsin and Road America. This was a moment I'd waited for, a long ride that would hopefully lead to me being able to speak with my new coworkers. They hadn't heard me say much; on that first weekend at Indy, I didn't ask for help or assistance and just wandered from task to task. Maybe with fewer people in a confined space, like a car, I'd open up. It worked that way with USAC and SKUSA.

But the car ride to Wisconsin was a quiet one for me. I tried, but everyone else in the van knew one another very well, so the conversations were like complicated dances they knew the steps to, but I didn't. Each time I thought I had something to say, I waited too long, and the dance moved on without me.

When we got to the track, I attempted to assist Trent in getting items out of the transporter, but much like the dance, I stepped on toes. I helped with items that didn't require help, and when he *needed* help, I wasn't prepared. When the large rolling cabinet almost broke free, Trent said, "Way to keep a guy hanging!"

I thought IMS had a lot of cable and fiber that needed to be dropped, but nothing could prepare me for this four-mile road course. For this race, I'd be working with Kim and Derby, whose jobs were making sure the timing lines in the track were operational and connecting the timing lines to the boxes that capture and transmit the data.

I liked this task because I could walk the entire track. I put to use my photography skills, getting some amazing shots of the scenic facility, but when it came to speaking with Kim and Derby, well, silence reigned supreme.

"Try, Aaron, try," I kept telling myself, but I could never find a way. What could I say? I was new and wondering how to sound normal and interesting rather than quiet and snobbish in my silence. I had a sinking feeling that I was coming across the way I feared I would.

As we got to the backside of the track, past the infamous kink but before Canada Corner, Kim stepped through the fence to plug something into the line. When she came back, she started complaining of some extreme leg itching and burning. I looked through the fence and saw a green plant growing in a dense pattern. I used my Google searching skills and within minutes I told Kim, "I think you lost a match with the plant called stinging nettle."

Kim and Derby looked at me, and Derby said, "You talk!" She seemed happy that I did, and for the rest of that day I talked with the two of them. By day's end, they knew most of my life story. It's amazing how once I'm able to take that first dance step, things don't go as badly as I feared they would. It's also amazing how people end up being much less scary than I feared they'd be. To this day, the story of the stinging nettle is often brought up.

Bryan Howard would be flying in to flag the IndyCar race, but I had two days of Road to Indy competition to flag. This series featured the USF2000 drivers and the Indy Pro drivers; to make a baseball comparison, this was the minor-league level, the feeder divisions for IndyCar. It was my first time flagging big-car road-course racing, and it soon became natural not to be able to see the entire track. Unlike IndyCar, where Kyle calls the green, in these feeder series the starter has that authority. The first time I exclaimed, "Green, green, green!" on the radio as I waved the flag over the field brought a surge of adrenaline.

Bryan arrived on Saturday. He and I had chatted on Facebook a few times over the years. After my first day in the stand for the 500 practice in 2016, he messaged me to say, "That experience is much like Pringles; you can't just have one." When he found out I was doing the Silver Crown race at Phoenix in 2017, he provided some insight about the track and wished me the best. He didn't know that we'd met in passing when I had Duane Sweeney re-sign my flag all those years ago, but when I brought it up at Road America, he remembered that day. As with Kim and Derby and the stinging nettles, that flag story got me into the conversational dance with Bryan.

Two other things stick out in my memory of that weekend. The first was the food. I probably spent way too much money, but the food served at a stand across from the flagstand was something I'd expect from a AAA five-diamond restaurant. The rib-eye sandwich? Savory, juicy, and filling for just $12, and it came with ice cream and a slice of pie baked by some church ladies. Sadly, the following year, both of these items disappeared. I still mourn this loss.

The second and more relevant memory is that on a mid-race restart, the heat shield on our communications box flew off from the immense aerodynamic turbulence generated by the passing cars. It blew up into the air and onto the race track. This heat shield was an extremely light, foil-like piece, but nonetheless I knew I had to radio it in.

What to say? How to say it? I started with, "Starter to control."

Jim responded, "Go ahead, starter."

My words had to be precise, quick, and delivered with confidence. "Yes, we've had an item, a heat shield, get blown off our radio case, and it's now on the track."

Jim responded, "Copy that, an item from the stand has blown onto the track."

A few seconds later, Kyle Novak was on the radio, asking, "Starter, what exactly is it?"

Kyle has a deep, booming voice, and had he not gone into race officiating he could've had a career as a narrator. But in a moment like this, that voice was intimidating. I did my best to describe the heat shield, and then he asked, "Do we need to go down for it?"

Down would be a full-course yellow. He was asking for my recommendation. The thing couldn't have been more than an ounce or two, as light as paper, really, so I said we could stay green. We did display the debris flag, but one of the cars clipped the shield and it was torn into a thousand pieces. The race went on.

I'm not sure if I was requested, but I was paired with Kim and Derby at teardown. I did my best at coiling the thousands of feet of fiber. I still wasn't fully competent, but I know my help was appreciated. More conversations were had, too. Maybe I was starting to step lightly into this dance of socializing.

Taking Flight in Iowa

IN THE MARATHON SUMMER OF 2020, THE NEXT EVENT WAS an oval doubleheader at Iowa Speedway, a pair of 250-lappers on Saturday and Sunday. For this event, we'd be flying to Des Moines from Indianapolis, and it would be my first time flying since the pandemic took hold.

Travel is something I've always enjoyed, to the point that I wrote a travel book that I never published. Anyway, the mood at an airport has always seemed festive to me, and I love everything about it. This time, however, there was a sense of dread in the air as I walked through the airport. Everyone seemed to have the same attitude.

I wondered to myself if contracting COVID was a guarantee. Masks were required, obviously, but was that enough? I did my best to avoid others, and others seemed to be doing the same. Gone was the festive atmosphere, and for me it was replaced with a haze of loss that hung in the air, like at a funeral. The joys of travel and the excitement of the next destination was lost to the great fear of the unknown. From Indy we flew to Chicago O'Hare, where the atmosphere was bleaker still. All the travelers stayed within their own packs, whether families or fellow workers, and it was eerily quiet, like a library. Once in Des Moines and out of the airport, it felt as if we'd jumped over a giant hurdle and broken free. For me, the sense of dread was replaced by the anticipation of seeing a new track.

Setup time at an oval is much quicker than at a road course. Once again, I was paired with Kim and Derby, who started asking more and more questions. I knew there had been some strong reservations about me after the first race, but those were fading. I felt more comfortable with my co-workers, and I think they began to see I did have a person-ality. It also helped that I was now candid about my autism, and the way it impacts me. Being so open wasn't a strong suit of mine, and still isn't, but I'm amazed at how much good it does for all parties involved.

Tom would be the number-one starter in this race, but he said that I'd be up front for a portion of it, just to get me more experience. This was going to feel a bit foreign to me. I had backed up Tom for a full decade, and now, sometime during this race, he would be helping me as I got some time at the helm.

Indy Cars on this 7/8-mile oval are spectacularly quick—the pole time was 18.371 seconds—so the race was flying by. Then, just past halfway, Will Power lost a left-front wheel shortly after a pit stop. The loose wheel bounced over the car, almost touching IndyCar's new Aeroscreen, designed to in-crease driver safety in these open-cockpit cars. This was nearly the Aeroscreen's first in-race crash test … and we wouldn't have to wait long for the real thing.

Tom gave me the nod when we got word that we'd be

going green next time by. This would be my first restart in IndyCar. But as the field entered turn three, I sensed trouble; I'd seen this scenario many times. The field was strung out and haphazard, and when this happens, you'll sometimes have cars in the back going faster than those ahead of them. I had a feeling this restart would be called off, and sure enough Jim announced, "No start. Yellow, yellow. No start." Tom had the yellow, so I backed away from the front of the stand.

The risk with wave-offs is that some drivers get the message, and some don't. The leaders slowed, and others further down in the order slowed, but some were still on the throttle. When Simon Pagenaud slowed, the trailing car of Rinus VeeKay slowed, but the slowdown happened too fast for Colton Herta to react. Colton hit the rear of Rinus's car, sending him skyward.

I wasn't expecting to see the undertray of an IndyCar, much less one headed in the direction of the flagstand. Once again, time slowed down, and life went frame-by-frame. I looked to be sure that Tom had the yellow, and I remember hoping that Colton's car did not get into the catch fence; it actually did graze the catch fence, but the car settled down trackside. He landed about 25 feet before the stand, and his car slid past us. Thankfully, as the AMR Safety Team got to him, he was unbuckling and uninjured after his scary flight. The good news was that as Colton's car climbed over Rinus's, the Aeroscreen on Rinus's car seemed to help deflect Colton's car up and away from Rinus's helmet.

I waved the green on the next restart, which was clean, and that evening Simon Pagenaud notched an incredible victory despite having started last, in the 23rd spot.

The next night, Tom had me do most of the race. Looking back, it felt natural to gain this type of experience a little at a time. I think it kept my nerves steady. At the time, I was a bit confused as to why we were swapping the flagging duties back and forth during the races; I worried that it was a lack of faith in my abilities. But flagging races in IndyCar—or any top series—carries immense pressure, and maybe the best way to learn to handle that pressure is to take it on gradually, a little at a time.

And speaking of pressure, the next event on the calendar was the 104th running of the Indianapolis 500.

The Month of May in August

IT WASN'T ON MEMORIAL DAY WEEKEND, BUT THERE WAS going to be an Indianapolis 500 run in its normal format, with a week of practice, a qualifying weekend, the traditional Carb Day final practice, and then race day. Sure, it was going to feel strange running it in August. But the biggest change was going to be on the other side of the catch fence. This would be a non-spectator event; the stands would be devoid of fans as the COVID-19 pandemic continued onward.

This was only my fourth IndyCar event, but I was finding my rhythm in the behind-the-scenes dance. I mostly knew which wires attached to which ends, and I lowered my expectations to where I was comfortable with on-the-job learning. That was a big problem I'd always had, this notion that I had to know everything right away or I was a failure. That was unrealistic. Besides, I was hired primarily as a flagman, and the job included lending assistance elsewhere when I could. I wasn't expected to know every last thing about a CAT5 communications cable, or how fiber optics work. But I was putting in the effort, not giving up, and learning.

I was also learning the ins and outs of the Speedway grounds. For example, I knew my way around the first two floors of the pagoda. Each time I walked past a patrolling yellow-shirted guard, I was sure I was going to be sent away. It just didn't seem possible that the same doors I'd regarded as forbidden were now mine to use.

I'd be the only starter on practice days. On the first day, Judge Boles, an observer in the stand, introduced himself. I told him that we'd worked together before, and he got a gigantic smile when he realized that I was that guy from 2016, and that I was now living my dream and fulfilling a destiny that started with Duane Sweeney's flag.

Each day of practice was a treat, but a bigger treat was just talking with Judge and trying to absorb all the history he shared. He told me about Duane, and what he was like on the stand, and he even had some insights on the Pat Vidan era. The hours shared with Judge that year, and in subsequent years, were a real blessing.

For qualifying, Tom and I split the duties, and it was then that the strangeness of this 2020 started to hit home. Tom mentioned frequently that, while it was still qualifying for the biggest race in the world, there was a lack of electricity in the air. When Marco Andretti nabbed the pole, what would surely have been a loud roar from the crowd was replaced with a silent stillness. The Andretti family's Indy curse struck again, robbing Marco of the cheers he earned.

I flagged Carb Day, and it was a shock to hear Bob Jenkins mention my name over the public-address system. I was a lifelong fan of Bob's announcing, and as a kid it was a dream to have him say my name as I was winning a major race somewhere. I wasn't winning a race on this day, but to have him say my name at IMS was an honor.

Now it was race day, but there weren't hundreds of thousands of fans rushing in to live a day of speed, tradition, and thrills. It felt surreal to drive to the track without a slowdown. On a normal race day, a late start leaving for the track might strand you in traffic for hours, but this was a straight shot.

Everything about this day was off somehow. It was still the Indianapolis 500, and whichever driver won would still be on the list of champions that will forever be remembered. But it felt more like *a* 500, not *the* 500.

I had resigned myself to the fact that I'd be on tablet duty, keeping track of the running order. Both Bryan and Tom were there, so they'd have the flagging more than handled. I did get interviewed that morning by a local Indy station; at one point, the lady interviewer asked, "What's it called, where you flag from? Is it the flag bucket?" Thanks to her, we do sometimes call it flag bucket now.

Pre-race ceremonies were … *different*. The best-attended sporting event in the world had no spectators, minus one guy who built a treehouse with a view from outside turn three. Despite the weird feeling, I still shed a few tears listening to "Back Home Again in Indiana."

The race started and the action on the track proved it was still *the* 500. Every driver had worked his entire career to be out there, and all 33 of them had every intention of being the first one across the bricks after 200 laps. I, too, had worked my entire career to be there, up in that flagstand, but I didn't want to get overly excited. I was the backup's backup. Still impressive, but I knew I'd have a chance someday.

A couple of yellow flags into the race, on the one-to-green lap, Bryan Howard said on the intercom, "You're up!" Wait, what? I said, "Up where?"

He turned, smiled, and said "Up here!"

There was no time to ask if he was sure. The field was headed for turn three, coiled for the restart. Moments later, Kyle Novak, full of energy, said, "GREEN! GREEN! GREEN!" I was restarting the Indianapolis 500!

It's hard to describe what that moment was like. I had no

time to prepare; it was reminiscent of the way my father almost tricked me into making my first presentation way back in 2009. The only thing that mattered was the task at hand.

As the last car flashed by, I put the green in the holder and started to inch back. Bryan asked, "Where are you going? You're still up!"

By race's end, I had done several restarts and had been up front for over half the race. As the race ended with Takuma Sato the winner, Tom Hansing finally got to wave the double checkered flags over the field. He had been the assistant starter for many years, and I could see in his face the joy this brought him.

I could talk or write all day about the 2020 Indianapolis 500, but this isn't where this story ends. I wasn't quite the chief starter of the race, like Duane Sweeney was. But my time would come.

A Season's End

IT HAD BEEN A BLUR. BEFORE I KNEW IT, THE INDYCAR season was coming to an end where it was supposed to have begun, in St. Petersburg. I had been at the SKUSA event in New Orleans when that St. Pete race was called off. I never could've envisioned the season that was to follow.

I had found my place within the setup-and-teardown team. Did I know how to do everything? Most certainly not, but I had become Trent's assistant, proficient at reading the fiber paperwork and taking notes for him. Google Earth also became my friend, and I premeasured a lot of the cable runs we did. It was a good way to be better prepared.

On the social front, I'd developed the ability to converse with everyone on the team. Along the way there were many team stories, like the time I tried a new energy-drink flavor and found it so repulsive that I spat it out of the van as we headed to Mid-Ohio. I've mentioned having to learn the dance steps I was ignorant of when I first came around; well, if someone new had come in at the end of 2020, they surely would've looked at me as if I'd known all the steps forever. This was fantastic and unexpected. So often in life I would not allow the time for relationships to develop, but when your life's passion brings you new people, you socialize.

With the season ending, however, a great deal of anxiety descended upon me. Would this be the end? Would I be invited back? Those were irrational fears that had no basis in reality, no evidence that pointed to that. One of the things that amplified these feelings was the retirement of the second scorer, Carla. I hate change, and the emotions I saw between Sharon and Carla were strong. I believe they'd worked decades together. I was still new to IndyCar, but to see someone decide that it was time to retire—that was hard for me. It made me think of all the people I had worked with, and all the people I had yet to work with, and I wrote this:

"What we owe to those we knew:

"Today was the final race of the NTT IndyCar season and the end of my first season. I could write about how exciting it's all been, but I learned something much more important this evening ...

"A person long involved in motorsports worked her last race today. I've only known her for not even four months, and in that time, I was so concerned about not screwing anything up. Actually, being so nervous to begin with made me blind to the fact that the timing team IndyCar has is filled with amazing people on and off the track. These nerves often prevent me from knowing others beyond the work they do. No one ever gets to truly know me, nor do I get to know them.

"A season's end, though … it's always emotional, and throw the year 2020 into the mix and it was already going to be extra emotional. Also, and I'm proud of myself on this, I have been coming out of my shell the past four events. I was getting to know the crew, and my personality was coming through after hiding under the 50,000-foot-deep shell I live under. However, the words I heard tonight shattered me: 'Good luck, and I'm glad I got to know you.'

"Time is hard for me to understand. I want everything to remain like it is right now, without change. Impossible, I know, but change is too often bad. Change is inevitable, but when it hits you in the face with such honest and emotional words it stings. I was the newbie, and this person went out of her way to give me something to hydrate after a hot day. But her words, that one sentence that ended with "know you," also gave me motivation to write this.

"What does this mean? What do we owe to those we come across like this in life? I say dedication; dedication to be just as awesome as those who came before us. Motorsports has been a thing since 1894. There have been many people who have started and ended careers, and there will be many, many more after us, and with each generation the lessons learned, the dedication, and the knowledge are passed on. This has created a lineage of officials that in one way does date all the way back to the creation of the sport itself. Granted, with each decade and evolution of the sport, skill sets have changed, but one thing that never has changed is the dedication people have for this sport. Today, a person's 40-year journey in the sport came to an end, and yet she told me those words I'll never forget, and for that I'm grateful. I'm actually brought to tears by those words for two reasons; the first is the sheer kindness of them; secondly, because I know someday, I'll be in that position. Hopefully it's a long way off, but there will be a time when I just won't be able to do it, and when that time comes, there may be a newbie on the team. Maybe they're

timid, like I was, and unsure of themselves. Maybe they've landed their dream gig, and, like me, they've got dedication to the sport without the ability to socialize. When that time comes, I'll remember tonight … and without any show of emotion I'll proudly let them know that I was happy to know them because I must be dedicated to the example set by those that paved the path before I came along."

That evening, as Scott Dixon and Chip Ganassi Racing celebrated the 2020 IndyCar championship, I was left wondering what the following season would hold for me. It felt like the end of the 2004 SLKA season. This made me smile because it put the entire journey together. The passion I had was the same back then as it was now. My path had been unbelievable so far, but destiny was going to be fulfilled in 2021.

——— The Road to the Finish Line ———

ANY WORRIES I HAD ABOUT NOT RETURNING IN 2021 WERE unfounded, because I most certainly was brought back for my second season as an IndyCar starter. The season began at Barber Motorsports Park, and I have to say, if you ever get the chance to visit Barber, you should go just to see the landscaping alone. The place is incredible! After that we went to St. Petersburg, and having closed the 2020 season there, it felt like we'd just left.

My first race as primary starter was part of a double-header at Texas Motor Speedway, another track that makes you say, "Wow!" Because of the banking, when you look towards turns three and four the cars are essentially at eye level. The skill the drivers have to use there can't really be translated on television; the speed, the banking, and the closeness of the racing make it a track that doesn't have many rivals when it comes to hair-raising excitement.

Once those early rounds were over, it was time to be, yes, back home again in Indiana, where I would be flagging the GMR Grand Prix on the road course to start the month of May.

Up to this point, I'd flagged many types of vehicles at many tracks, but now I was flagging—not just assisting—at the Indianapolis Motor Speedway. Sure, I'd had my stint as the starter "up front" at the 500 in August of 2020, but that wasn't quite the same. After all, I didn't know it was happening until it was happening, in mid-race. And, of course, there were no spectators. Now, in 2021, the electricity was back at IMS, and as Rinus VeeKay won the Grand Prix I did a little pointing/stopping motion with my flags. Track photographer Walter Kuhn got an amazing shot of this, and I had no idea what that little movement with the flags would lead to.

Once again, I would flag practice solo, and this year Bryan Howard and I would do qualifying.

Oval-track qualifying wasn't something I had much experience doing. When I flagged as a child atop that rock on the side of my street, I would often emulate Duane Sweeney's qualifying style. But when I tried it in the stand in 2020, it just didn't feel right for me. I thought it was fine, but that style belonged to Duane; I had to find my own. Trent kept telling me, "Aaron, every starter here has had a signature move, what's yours?" I wasn't looking for a signature move; I found that the best way to find a signature move was by accident.

I may sound like a "flag nerd" here, and it's hard to describe certain movements on paper. But halfway through a practice session, I started slashing the flag downward, and I liked that. Then I began "following" a car with the flag horizontal, pointing at it as it sped away toward turn one, and added a tiny freeze for drama. In some sensory way, my body loved this motion. When I flagged on that rock as a boy, it wasn't just that I enjoyed moving the flag through the air as cars went by; there was a positive physical sensation. I felt that again in the IMS flagstand as each car went by and I rotated my body to bring the flag towards turn one. It was euphoric!

I wasn't the only one enjoying this accidental, newfound style. Videos started popping up on social media, and it seemed to be a hit. No one knew my name until Dave Furst, IndyCar's vice president of communications, tweeted a video he shot from pit lane. Dave mentioned that he enjoyed the added flair because, after all, it's Indy.

Spectator after spectator stopped me to say they loved the flag show. I never thought of what I did as being something fans would enjoy; I just liked flagging and having a role in the races. As you must know by now, when those on the autism spectrum are doing something within "their Kansas," it's because they enjoy it. Yes, I wanted it to look good, but I never imagined it would lead a person to offer a positive comment.

I look back at all the hurdles I had to jump, all the adversity I faced, and it was the passion for motorsports that allowed me to persevere. From the issues I had in school, to more recent things with my job, each event had the potential to destroy me. But now my passion was on display, and people were enjoying it.

After qualifying, I treated Bryan to dinner at Noble Roman's on 10th Street, the same place I was when I had texted Doug Boles five years prior to get that one day of practice. I felt like it was only right to show Bryan where my IndyCar journey began. We talked about history, about Duane Sweeney, and about tracks no longer in existence.

I assumed the 500 would be Bryan's to flag, because I had done the Grand Prix. But out of nowhere, his face got solemn and he put down his pizza.

He said, "Aaron, we need to talk."

Naturally, I panicked, fearing that somehow he'd learned that I was being fired.

"I've watched you grow this past year," said Bryan. "You've become so much more confident in all that you're doing, in and out of the stand. So, I have to ask, do you want the 500 from start to finish? Are you ready?"

Imagine that moment. Try to freeze time and process what I just heard. Think about a lifetime of work, a lifetime of heartbreaks, a lifetime of closed doors that somehow opened up into incredible possibilities. This moment was a culmination of everything on these pages, as well as events I haven't written about. This was everything I wanted, everything I dreamed of.

I know it must have sounded like a cliché, but I meant it when I told Bryan, "I've been ready for this since Duane gave me his checkered flag."

The 500

THE BIG WEEKEND CAME, AND WITH IT CAME A NEED TO warm up. Carb Day had been extremely cold, but my heart was warmed by fans who said they loved my work. As the videos circulated, it slowly became public knowledge that I was on the autism spectrum. WTHR, the NBC affiliate in Indianapolis, asked if they could interview me at my first flagstand, the rock in my childhood neighborhood. Rich Nye, "the Sports Guy," came out to do the interview. It was fun to see the current residents of our old cul-de-sac walk out looking rather confused; why was a rock at the edge of their world creating so much attention? In the end, they thought it was cool that the flagman for the Indianapolis 500 got his start right there, on that rock.

The night before the race, I had dinner with my dad, who was naturally in town for the race. The dinner was rather quiet. I don't know how drivers handle the stress before the 500, because I was locked up emotionally. There were so many things I wanted to say; I wanted to thank my dad for all the sacrifices of money and time. But I was busy fending off pressure that had my entire body wanting to cease all movement. Was there a hole I could crawl into and hide? No amount of preparation could prepare me for this night. The big things going through my mind were, "Don't screw up" and "Don't drop a flag!" Two simple tasks yet, on a stage like the Indianapolis 500, the pressure is unmeasurable. Somehow, I ate enough to squash my hunger, and then it was time to sleep, to rest up for tomorrow.

Because tomorrow, destiny would be fulfilled.

To beat the race-day traffic, staff is encouraged to get to the track before 5:00 a.m. At that hour, on that day, the Speedway grounds are full of potential energy on the brink of becoming the most beautiful and contagious energy in the world. I could feel it as I drove in through the tunnel off of 16th Street. I had done this many times, but this time the emotions spilled out. I cried. I cried a lot. It was overwhelming, thinking back to the winding road that had been my journey. I then got choked up thinking of those who were no longer here. I'd have given anything to just let them know what their part in this journey meant to me.

It was a strange reaction, right then, to have this sense of regret at my inability to thank people in my life. I thought back to when Carla had retired from the scoring staff, and the piece I'd written for myself on the emotions of that happening. I thought about the night of my diagnosis, so many years ago, and how I had thought my life would come down to this: No friends, no job, no happiness.

That now made me laugh. I had established many meaningful connections with others, in my own way. Sure, if you judge these things by the way "normal" people interact, then okay, maybe I never had a meaningful connection. But I believe the relationships I have mean more to me than the relationships shared by many "normal" people. Expressing the meaning of this, and the emotions attached to it, is a weak point of mine. But as I got out of the car on the morning of the 105th Indianapolis 500, I knew I had triumphed over the nonsense I had read on the night of my diagnosis, and the outlook it gave me for so long.

Being at the track so early leads to quite a waiting game. I took many photos of the sunrise while bouncing around the property like a 5-year-old on Red Bull, and this diversion also helped me stay ahead of the pressure. Again, I have no idea how the 33 drivers in the race handle this; unlike them, I wouldn't be traveling at 230 miles per hour, inches away from other cars whose drivers all had the same mission: to win the 500 by taking calculated risks.

As the morning crept on, Jon Koskey introduced me to actor Milo Ventimiglia, star of "The Art of Racing in the Rain," who would be serving as honorary starter. Milo was amazingly gracious towards me, especially considering that I had a partial shutdown because of the flurry of people around him. We talked briefly about his duties, the basics of which were: "Wave the green when I tap you on the shoulder, and, above all else, don't drop the flag. That is not something you want to be immortalized for."

I was able to spend some personal time with my dad. Even though I was now an official, this was still a day steeped in tradition, and so much of that involved us being together. Sure, my "seat" was going to be much better than his now, but I still wanted to experience the atmosphere of the day with him. As much as that day was marked by me reaching the summit after climbing a steep mountain, it was also a moment of celebration for my dad. For the race, he would be seated across the track, just north of victory lane. I wouldn't be able to see him, because the colors and faces in a crowd that big tend to blur. But he'd be able to see me for the entire race.

When 11:00 a.m. came, I said goodbye to my dad and walked to the base of the flagstand. I could feel my pulse in every corner of my body. The reality of what I was about to do was hammered home when a fan approached me and opened an autograph book. He said he'd been coming to the race for 51 years, and he wanted my autograph. I froze when he pointed for me to sign at a spot between legendary journalist Chris Economaki and Jim Nabors, the longtime singer of "Back Home Again in Indiana." Who was I compared to them? Look, anyone can wave a flag, and perhaps someday the flags at race tracks will be a thing of the past, totally replaced by lights. I asked this man several times if he was sure that's where he wanted me to sign. He nodded and said, "It's been a long time since there was style like you have. Besides, you're the eighth chief starter of the race!" With that, I signed his book and looked up at the flagstand, awed by the idea that my autograph rested between the signatures of those two legends.

Milo Ventimiglia and his entourage made it to the base of the stand, and we waited there; the stand was occupied at the moment by Indiana Army National Guard bugler Ron Duncan, who played "Taps." I was nervous, and I think Milo picked up on that, because he looked down and complimented me on my choice of footwear. It was just a little thing, but it lessened my nerves. Also, his grace with the adoring fans gathered at the fence was calming.

With each tick of the clock, the reality of what was about to take place grew more vivid. I had imagined this moment forever. How could I cope with the emotions and the pressure at the same time? As if to add even more weight, Jim

Swintal in race control gave a last pre-race radio instruction to those working the race: "The eyes of the racing world are watching us today. Let's take care of each other, do a lot of good. God bless and see you on the flip side."

It was time to ascend the ladder for the final time this May.

Rung by rung I climbed. Emotions were thick, memories swirling, but as I reached the top of the flagstand there was a sense of clarity. This was it! This was the Indianapolis 500! The lingering COVID restrictions may have capped the crowd at 135,000, but this was the real thing. As I surveyed the cars, the crowd, and the flags awaiting me, I knew I had a job to do, and there would be no failing at this.

In all the years I'd attended the race as a fan, the minutes between the national anthem and the singing of "Back Home Again in Indiana" were the longest in sports. Now, standing in the 34th-best seat at the track, it was an eternity. I couldn't help but think of everyone I knew. I wondered if any of my old classmates knew I was doing this; they sure got annoyed when I would talk about this track, this race, and the flags for hours on end, but look where I was now! Did the people I raced against have any idea? Did Frankie Neidenbach's family know about this? I remembered the first time I handed Frankie a flag. How could anyone have imagined that would lead to this? My smile was interrupted as photographer Walter Kuhn snapped some photos of me with Milo. Unashamedly, I then took a photo of my own, a selfie with Milo.

Then came the introduction of Jim Cornelison and the Purdue University All-American Marching Band, and the opening notes to "Back Home Again in Indiana."

Tears. Lots and lots of tears flowed. Don't let anyone tell you that a person on the autism spectrum can't be emotional. All the emotions connected to the 500—races past, and races to come—overwhelmed me. I did what I could to hide my tearful emotions from Milo, because who wants to cry in front of a celebrity, let alone the honorary starter?

As the sound of the second military flyover faded into the skies south of the track, Roger Penske's voice echoed around the track on the public-address system:

"Drivers, start your engines!"

The sound of 33 engines and the cheers of thousands filled the most famous straightaway in racing. When I heard Jim Swintal in my headset saying, "Pace car, roll out," I picked up the yellow flag and displayed it vertically. This was it. The race cars were in motion, and we would be going green on their fourth trip past the flagstand.

Minutes later, the field passed beneath us. Jim Swintal said, "Pace car, that was first time by."

Next: "Pace car and starter, that was the second time by."

And then: "Pace car and starter, this is one to green." I gave the one-to-green signal, just like I had at so many Quarter Midget races. This, of course, was a slightly bigger deal.

I handed Milo Ventimiglia the flag, and asked if he had any final questions. He had been terrific the entire time and was just as eager and excited as I was, but he said he was ready. The field, in 11 rows of three, were on the backstretch.

I listened to race control: "Starter, the field is in turn three, stand by … field is in four …"

I saw the front row: Scott Dixon on the pole, Colton Herta in the middle, Rinus VeeKay outside.

"Stand by, starter … GREEN, GREEN, GREEN!"

I tapped Milo on the shoulder. He did a decent job with the green flag. Suddenly, a mad pack of cars stormed under us, running so tightly together that the colors blended together. When Colton Herta took the lead on the backstretch, the crowd erupted in cheers.

As strong as my emotions had been before the race, they evaporated with the start. All the spectators disappeared, too. Nothing registered with me now but the cars and race control.

After several laps, as things settled down, we said good-bye to Milo. He said, "I may have been in a lot of shows, but you have the best job in the world!"

I smiled, and thought: If you only knew the entire story …

With the first round of pit stops came the day's first incident. Stefan Wilson's car locked its brakes as he entered pit lane; I saw it jump sideways and make contact with the wall. I had the yellow flag ready and *almost* threw it too soon but held it. Right away, however, came the call: "Pits are closed, pits are closed. Yellow, yellow!"

After the restart came a long stretch of green flag racing that took us well past the halfway point. I kept my attention on the track, but somewhere in the back of my mind was a faint montage of memories: coming to the track as a young boy, reacting to the volume of the engines, insisting on staying there despite the pain from that noise. What if my dad had never brought me here? I looked across the track and smiled; he was one of the faces in that crowd. There were memories, too, of Duane Sweeney and his flag. I'd have given anything to be able to tell him all the things I should have said in that thank-you note I never wrote. And Ron Ekstrand; would I have ever developed the confidence to do my work in front of millions if not for the speaking opportunities he gave me? What about all of the people, friends and strangers alike, who advocated for me when the starter's job opened up at IndyCar?

If there's a lesson in my story, it's that those on the spectrum, if given the chance, can do amazing things. I was horrible at networking, I was horrible at interviewing, and at every job I had it took me a long while to feel comfortable. But the jobs themselves? Once I figured them out, I was more than able. You can't fake passion, and if you're capable at a job and your passion shows through, hopefully people notice that like they noticed it in me.

Judge Boles was with us on the stand as an observer, and

on lap 119 he stomped his feet. A fraction of a second later, race control called for the yellow flag. Coming out of the pits after a stop, Graham Rahal, who'd been in contention for the win, lost a wheel and spun in front of a fast-approaching train of cars. It was a scary incident that could have involved many cars, but Rahal was the only one eliminated.

Alex Palou led the field on the restart, followed by Helio Castroneves, who was looking to become just the fourth driver to win four Indy 500s. Before they reached turn one, Helio took the lead, to the delight of the crowd. The remaining race between Castroneves, Palou, and Pato O'Ward will become part of the Speedway's legend.

The laps began to dwindle. There was a time when the late stages of the Indianapolis 500 were the saddest minutes of the year for me, because they marked the beginning of a long wait until the next year's race. This time, though, I was focused only on *this* 500. It would end with me throwing the double checkered flags. My heart rate picked up.

With seven laps to go, Takuma Sato, the two-time and defending race winner, pitted from the lead. Seconds later, Castroneves swept around Palou and took the lead. The roar from the crowd nearly drowned out the engines. A win by Helio would tie him with A.J. Foyt, Al Unser Sr., and Rick Mears. History was at hand.

When I put my hand out to show five laps to go, Palou pulled the same move Helio had made on him, and now Alex had the lead.

The anticipation from the crowd was immense. I could feel it from the stand. As the leaders completed lap 198, race control was in my ear: "Starter, white flag next time." Helio chose that very moment to slingshot around Alex, and now he was in front. The anticipation became a frenzy. I couldn't hear the cars anymore.

Would Palou get him back? The leaders had caught up with a dense pack of slower cars. The pink-and-black car of the leader, Castroneves, was actually seventh in line, with Palou's blue-and-white car on his tail. To complicate things, there was another pink-and-black car in that group. If the timing of the checkered flags was off by a car or two in that line, it wouldn't change the finish, but it would take away from the moment, and perhaps ruin the traditional shot of the finish. Nerves? Oh, yeah, there were nerves.

The string of cars exited turn four. I waved the white flag over Helio and Alex, and then conscious breathing ceased. Bryan called for me to hand off the white, so I could grab the two checkered flags. With the leaders on the backstretch still facing heavy traffic, I watched the video screen, hoping that there'd be some separation of the cars, but there was none.

Off of turn four they came for the final time. I looked for Helio's pink-and-black car and found it. As he approached the line, I began a wave that was 38 years in the making; in other words, all my life. The timing was perfect, and as the last of the top five cars passed by, I did the brief freeze, which even showed up on the NBC telecast. As more cars completed the race, I continued to wave with every ounce of passion I had. When the last cars had passed, my flags pointed them toward turn one as they disappeared.

And then I could breathe.

The roar of the crowd would not die down. The people knew what was next. As Helio finished his victory lap, he parked just past the yard of bricks, climbed from the cockpit, and went to his own signature move, climbing the catch fence. His team followed suit. The roar of the crowd was unlike anything I'd ever heard.

I looked down on the celebration for several seconds, but then turned my gaze across the frontstretch and pit lane, to the section where my dad was seated. I smiled and, once again, teared up.

History will record this as Helio's day. Somewhere, maybe, my name will appear in a note recording who was chief starter.

But for me, personally, it was a day for every person who gave me a chance, had faith in me, allowed me to feel comfortable and grow, and supported me in the work I did. This day was for Matt, for Kyle, for Ron, James, Jon, and all the rest, going back to my very first job.

And this day was for my dad, who got to see me do the impossible. Impossible stories are what make the Indianapolis 500 so great, so legendary. I'm just a small part of that, but for me, the impossible did happen.

As the crowd continued to roar, I looked to the sky and said, "Thank you," to all who were here, and to all who weren't.

What We Can Learn from
Playing in Traffic

Paula Pompa-Craven, PsyD
Easterseals Southern California
easterseals.com/southerncal

THERE ARE SO MANY ILLUSTRATIVE POINTS IN THIS BOOK, lessons to learn, struggles and important messages of support and success. Simply put, autistic/neurodiverse individuals can and are doing great things and living fulfilling lives. Here are just a few themes reflected in this book for consideration:

Why this book is important:

This is a book about hope, how important it is to have it, and what happens when it is lost. Studies of learned hopefulness theory suggest that those experiences that allow us to build skills and to develop a sense of control are empowering. This sense of empowerment brings hope and reduces the negativity one might be experiencing or feeling. Hopefulness leads to happiness and can lead to success. At the age of 20, Aaron reports that he had "given up hope of working, hope of contributing to the world, hope of normal everyday relationships. I'd given up hope, period." (p.3) He later talks about offering hope (p.146) and the hope that he brings to others during his presentations to officers with children with ASD (p.191). Aaron later summarizes his hope as he reports, "I smiled and thought back to that parent-training program, and I said, 'Yes, I still want to race, but it's a new race now. I didn't know it for most of my life, but there is so much hope for those on the autism spectrum…but only if society is aware of its existence'" (p.182). This is the type and level of hope that motivates forward movement and leads to a higher quality of life.

The evolution of a diagnosis:

The Diagnosis of Autism Spectrum Disorder (ASD) has evolved and its prevalence has increased dramatically. When Aaron was diagnosed, late in life, the incidence was 1 in 125; today it is 1 in 36 per the CDC. When Aaron was diagnosed with Asperger's Syndrome, which is now part of the autism umbrella (pp.27, 102), often referring to himself as an "Aspie" (p.3), he suffered from a major failure by the diagnosing doctor, "I really don't know what to say. Good luck?" Today, the information, resources and services available to people have advanced considerably. Our language has changed, and there is health insurance coverage across the country to support people with ASD. Most importantly, there is a push to change our communities and practices to provide access for, and acceptance of, the nuances of people with ASD rather than changing autistic people to fit into our communities. Understanding the incidence of ASD and the importance of early diagnosis and support is key. People tend to get information or misinformation from various places that could lead to misperceptions and misunderstandings (p.193). It is important to get information from reliable sources. (See for example, https://www.easterseals.com/southerncal .) During one of Aaron's presentations, a student simply stated, "Isn't autism simply that you see and process the world around you differently?" (pp.215, 216). No judgment, just different.

The intersectionality of ASD and mental health:

Co-occurring diagnoses are extremely common for people with ASD. In fact, according to the National Institute of Health (NIH), between 73%-81% of adults have both a mental health and an autism diagnosis. These typically include anxiety and depression. Children with autism also may have ADHD, anxiety, depression, food and sleep disorders. All of these should be considered and addressed by a qualified mental health practitioner. Throughout Aaron's life he has described symptoms of anxiety including lots of school anxiety (pp.12-18, 84), work anxiety (pp.113, 138, 252) and depression (pp.29, 119, 242, 248, 252). At times, his depression was intense, keeping him in bed, leading to negative self-talk and defeatist thoughts. Therapy and ongoing psychological and psychiatric support can be beneficial. It is often difficult but important to find trained practitioners with the skill set to support.

Characteristics and myths about people with ASD:

There are a range of attributes associated with people with ASD that may result in a diagnosis, as demonstrated throughout the book. Aaron described many of the challenges or experiences that he faced. For example, there are several instances of difficulty with communication (pp.93-94, 171, 234), including struggles with non-verbal communication such as less eye contact (p.16) and trouble understanding non-verbal or social cues (pp.77, 191). Other characteristics include challenges with social/emotional reciprocity (pp.16, 109), including perspective-taking (pp.20-23, 29) and rigidity of thought (p.152). One example of rigidity of thought is Aaron's report of "whatever happens first always has to happen" (p.20). Other examples of characteristics include rule-governed behavior (pp.15-16) and delayed processing speed (pp.17, 94-95, 102, 171-172). There are many reports of sensory sensitivities, including to sound (p.17), food (p.207) and drums (p.244). There are also restricted interests about racing (p.8, 97), flags, (p.9) and many other topics.

It is important to recognize that while some of these challenges are characteristics used in diagnosing ASD, they are not all representative of autistic people. Some people associate these challenges with a lack a of empathy, love or feeling, which is not accurate. There are many times throughout the book that Aaron describes or provides contrary evidence to these myths (pp.76, 155, 241).

Strategies to Support & Uplift:

A key component of Aaron's successes throughout his life could be contributed to the number of strengths that he demonstrates, along with the support of family and friends. Something that these support people do, possibly without realizing it, is strength-spotting. Strength-spotting is the focus on strengths, rather than deficits to identify ways to increase confidence and support growth (pp.110, 117). This strength-based approach eventually led to Aaron's dream job. Also, some of his teachers used this technique, which was recognized by Aaron when he states, "Thank you for not just teaching me, but reaching me" (p.23). This is the goal for all the individualized support that should be provided to people with ASD. Also, it is wonderful to see how Aaron was able to turn what might at one time have been described as restricted patterns of interests, which others might describe as passion, into opportunities for employment. Through relationship-building, slowly but steadily, Aaron gains trust, skill, and learns to advocate for himself (p.220). Aaron shares his story, his struggles, his openness so that others might benefit. His trainings (p.236) might save lives. This book is a reminder of that and about how open communication leads to more inclusive practices (p.278). In Aaron's words, "If there's a lesson in my story, it's that those on the spectrum, if given the chance, can do amazing things" (p.295).

Testimonials

"Since meeting Aaron Likens in 2009 and hiring him as an Autism Ambassador, his impact has been profound. *Playing in Traffic* distills his incredible journey from living with an autism spectrum diagnosis to becoming an acclaimed flagman for the Indy 500 and a beacon of hope for countless individuals. Through his writing and his thousands of public presentations to a diverse array of audiences—from parents and educators to healthcare professionals, law enforcement, and even the FBI—Aaron has shared invaluable insights into life on the spectrum. His book is not just a story of racing or personal achievement; it's a road map for understanding and inclusion, demonstrating the immeasurable value of seeing the world through a different lens."
—*Ron Ekstrand, CEO Easterseals Arkansas*

"I picked Aaron to be the flagman for the SKUSA Super-Nationals because, quite frankly, he is the best flagman in the world. No doubt about it."
—*Tom Kutscher, SuperKarts USA*

"It's been a privilege to watch Aaron's life journey, both as a flagman and an inspirational speaker and educator in the field of autism awareness. His passion and dedication for motorsports flagging has been on display since his initial days in karting, and to see his supreme talent and laser focus on perfection rewarded and embraced with IndyCar is proof that good things do happen to good people."
—*Rob Howden, ekartingnews.com*

"In 2009, Aaron and his dad, Jim, walked into my office at the United States Auto Club. Aaron was quiet and reserved. Jim explained that Aaron had a condition that allowed him to process things visually more quickly than most people.

He'd always wanted to use those skills to follow his hero, Duane Sweeney, and be a flagman. Intrigued, I talked with James Spink, who headed up our .25 Midget program for youth racers, which is visually one of the fastest-moving series we have. I asked James to give Aaron a shot. After his third or fourth event, I overheard a young driver's father comment that 'this new flagman is the best we've ever had!' I'm very proud of Aaron, and inspired by his determination."
> *—Jason Smith, USAC, Sr. VP Race Operations*

"Whether it was a .25 Midget or a USAC Regional or National Midget race, I was happy to have Aaron waving the flags. His on-track work and dedication speak for themselves, but what impressed me most was his personal growth away from the tracks. We had a nucleus of young team members who enjoyed going out together for dinner, fun, and new adventures in the cities we travelled to. Seeing Aaron come out of his shell was fun to watch. He was one of us, and having him as part of our team made us better. I swear, in all my years of racing, he was the one flagman I never saw make a mistake!"
> *—James Coppola. USAC Developmental Series*
> *Director 2008-2012*

"I, as many others do, often think of driving a race car on the limit as a form of art. But, until I saw Aaron flag, I hadn't understood and appreciated the artistry possible in that position. I didn't think Pole Day at the Indy 500 could get any better, but from my new seat in the booth, on the 9th floor of the pagoda, I get an unobstructed view of Aaron performing his craft over and over, and it has brought even more joy to an already amazing day."
> *–James Hinchcliffe, NBC IndyCar broadcaster and*
> *former IndyCar driver*

Comments on Aaron Likens's Presentations to the Autism-Awareness Community:

"Never in my career have I seen one individual captivate our student body, share so much information in such a unique way, make students laugh and cry, and do it all in 19 minutes."
> —*Tim Detviler, Asst. Principal, Lutheran High School of Orange County*

"I cannot express our gratitude to Aaron for speaking at our symposium. The feedback that I have received supports his incredible gift to the audience with his personal reflection. He is truly a gift to the field. I feel very proud to have met him."
> —*Dr. Terrie Inder, Professor in Pediatrics, Neurology and Radiology, Washington University, St Louis, Missouri*

"Aaron Likens may be the most courageous, intelligent, and tenacious young man I have met in my long tenure in the mental health field. He is fiercely determined to better understand himself and the world around him, and he does us the great favor of sharing his journey of self-discovery, so profoundly touched by Asperger's Syndrome. We have much to learn from Aaron."
> —*Dr. Keith Schafer, Retired Director, Missouri Department of Mental Health*

"I wanted to let you know I was in attendance for Aaron Likens's presentation for our in-service training on Autism. Aaron was great!! I have been to a lot of trainings in my 37-year career and Aaron is one of the best speakers I have heard. Thank you for allowing us to use Aaron for this training."
> —*Sgt. Barry Armfield, St. Louis Area Crisis Intervention Team Coordinator (RET), St. Louis County Police Department*

"Aaron Likens's presentation was the best professional-development activity I have ever attended in my 25-plus years in education on any topic."
—*Mike Vaia, Special Services Director, Hannibal Public Schools, Hannibal, Missouri*

"Aaron Likens's presentation for our third to eighth graders was FANTASTIC. I've been in education for forty-six years and that was the best hour I have ever spent! His information was understandable for students and thought-provoking for our staff!"
—*William Unzicker, Lutheran School principal, Perryville, Missouri*

Index